LEARNING

HOW THE

HEART BEATS

*L*EARNING

HOW THE

HEART
BEATS

THE MAKING OF A
PEDIATRICIAN

CLAIRE McCARTHY, M.D.

VIKING

VIKING
Published by the Penguin Group
Penguin Books USA Inc., 375 Hudson Street,
New York, New York 10014, U.S.A.
Penguin Books Ltd, 27 Wrights Lane, London W8 5TZ, England
Penguin Books Australia Ltd, Ringwood, Victoria, Australia
Penguin Books Canada Ltd, 10 Alcorn Avenue,
Toronto, Ontario, Canada M4V 3B2
Penguin Books (N.Z.) Ltd, 182–190 Wairau Road,
Auckland 10, New Zealand

Penguin Books Ltd, Registered Offices:
Harmondsworth, Middlesex, England

First published in 1995 by Viking Penguin,
a division of Penguin Books USA Inc.

1 3 5 7 9 10 8 6 4 2

AUTHOR'S NOTE

The stories in this book are based on real events and people. The names
and certain identifying details of patients and their families have been
changed in order to protect their privacy.

Portions of this work first appeared in different form as a series of articles
in the *Boston Globe* magazine. The chapters "The Laying On of Hands"
and "Mouthing the Words" were previously published in *Hippocrates* magazine. A condensation of this book appeared in *Today's Best Nonfiction*,
published by Reader's Digest.

LIBRARY OF CONGRESS CATALOGING IN PUBLICATION DATA
McCarthy, Claire, M.D.
Learning how the heart beats: the making of a
pediatrician/Claire McCarthy.
p.   cm.
ISBN 0–670–83874–8
1. McCarthy, Claire, M.D.   2. Women pediatricians—United
States—Biography.   3. Pediatrics—Popular works.   I. Title.
RJ43.M33A3   1995
618.92'00092—dc20
[B]   94–11596

This book is printed on acid-free paper.

∞

Printed in the United States of America
Set in Minion
Designed by Ann Gold

For Mark, who makes my dreams possible,
and for Deborah,
who was too beautiful to be possible

I would like to thank Ande Zellman, who, as editor of the *Boston Globe Magazine,* gave me a chance and inspired me to keep writing. I would also like to thank Pamela Dorman, Paris Wald, and Carolyn Carlson, the editors at Viking Penguin who have worked on this book; their help has been invaluable.

Most of all, I would like to thank my agent, Doe Coover. Without her enthusiasm, her insight, and her steadfast support, this book would never have been written.

CONTENTS

INTRODUCTION

When I was an intern, working in the neonatal intensive care unit, I held a baby who had just died. He was born prematurely, and although we tried very hard, we couldn't save him. His parents had said their good-byes and given him to me to take away.

I cradled him in my arms, gently, almost afraid I might hurt him. I looked down at his tiny, blue face; his eyes were closed, and his delicate features were frozen in that last moment when his heart stopped beating. I kissed his forehead and laid him down softly in the bassinet, reflexively pulling up his blanket.

Mesmerized by his motionlessness, I stood there and stared at him. I didn't want to leave him alone. It was very quiet in the room, quieter than it had ever been before; even the noise from the busy intensive care unit next door seemed dulled and muffled. It was as if the air were filled with reverence, like the air in a church.

I didn't cry. I didn't think doctors were supposed to cry. But all of me wanted to cry, and I felt dazed and numb as

I walked home from the hospital. I was only vaguely aware of the cars whizzing by or the people around me. My feet found the curbs more out of habit than because I saw them.

As soon as I got to my apartment I sat down at my computer and began to write about the baby. Tomorrow his place in the unit would be taken; perhaps it already had been. There would be another sick baby to think about, and before long I would forget this one who had just died, or at least I would forget the details: his beautiful little eyes, his tiny, perfect hands, how he fought so hard for his life, and how his parents held him close as he died. I didn't want to forget, so I wrote it all down.

I wrote not just to remember, but to ease my sorrow, pain, and confusion. I always wrote when something upset or moved me. Putting events and emotions into words and then reading them, either right away or days or weeks later, made things more clear, more understandable, and less overwhelming.

As I went through medical training I spent a lot of time sitting at my computer late at night or curled up in bed with a notebook, writing until my fingers were sore. There were so many lives to be recorded, so many moments and details that were important to remember. There were so many times when writing was the only way I could sort through the issues and feelings and find some measure of peace.

The process of becoming a doctor took me seven years. Medical school was four years, and Harvard divided these into two parts. The first two years were spent attending lectures, doing laboratory exercises, and poring over textbooks, studying the science of the human body, its diseases and their treatment. We studied every blood vessel, bone, muscle, and nerve and learned about the function of every organ and system. We stared down microscopes until our eyes hurt, looking at slides of every tissue, bacterium, and parasite. We learned about everything that could possibly go wrong, how infection, injury, malformation, and cancer could affect the organs and systems. We learned so much that sometimes I thought there wasn't room in my brain for one more piece of information. It was hard work, but I loved it. Medicine was far and away the most interesting and important thing I had ever studied.

Thus armed with a basic understanding of medicine, we spent the second two years in the various hospitals associated with Harvard. We were divided into small groups and did "clerkships" in different areas of medicine such as internal medicine, surgery, pediatrics, obstetrics, gynecology, and radiology. Each clerkship was one to three months long. We were excited about these clerkships, since they allowed us to work with patients instead of books.

Some of the teaching in the clerkships was done in teaching sessions led by residents or senior physicians. They would go over diagnoses and treatments, give us copies of articles from medical journals, and quiz us, using the cases of real or imaginary patients. Most of the teaching, however, was done by involving the medical students as apprentices. We were assigned patients to care for, we took part in surgical operations, we attended rounds and were given whatever tasks the doctors felt would teach us more about their areas of medicine. We wore white coats and did our best to blend in and become essential parts of the medical team.

We were usually paired with interns and residents, whom we followed, worked with, and took overnight call with, who taught us the nuts and bolts of taking care of patients. They taught us how to write orders and progress notes, how to draw blood and put in IVs, how to know which problems could wait and which couldn't. Some went out of their way to include us whenever possible; others were less enthusiastic about teaching and often ignored us. But no matter what, we remained somewhat in awe of them for knowing what to do and being comfortable with it. Whatever time they spent with us, we learned from watching them—we learned how to act like doctors.

During the fourth year of medical school we had to decide which area of medicine we wanted to specialize in and apply to residency programs for that specialty. I chose pediatrics. I had actually chosen pediatrics when I was twelve years old, which was when I'd decided to be a doctor. Both at twelve and at twenty-four, my reasons for choosing pediatrics were not particularly complex; I liked being around children, and I thought that it was the area of medicine where I would be most happy.

I did my residency, which was three years long, at Children's Hospital in Boston. Children's is a large, tertiary-care referral center affiliated with Harvard University that offers everything for children from heart transplants to baby shots, from the latest in cancer treatments to evaluations of children with learning disorders. It serves patients from all over the world, as well as those from the local inner-city neighborhoods.

Although I was officially a doctor when I started my residency, I still had a lot to learn, especially about pediatrics. That's the way medical training works: medical school teaches us a great deal, but supervised experience is necessary before we can go out on our own.

I learned pediatrics the way I learned medicine during the last two years of medical school—as an apprentice, working under doctors senior to me. The other residents and I rotated through the different parts of the hospital. We spent time on the wards, taking care of children with almost every possible illness, from asthma to diabetes to AIDS. We worked in the intensive care units, taking care of critically ill children, many of them on ventilators and maximal life supports. We worked in the emergency room, the cardiology service, the cancer service, the bone marrow transplant unit, and the outpatient clinics. We saw patient after patient, worked very long hours, and took turns staying overnight in the hospital as often as every third night. It was not just an apprenticeship, it was learning by immersion.

We were the front line. We did the work of caring for patients: performing daily examinations, scheduling tests, hunting down results, dealing with seemingly endless paperwork, doing procedures such as IVs, responding to emergencies. Frequently sleep deprived, we were constantly being thrown into new situations, sometimes being given more responsibility than we thought we could handle. All of this left us feeling raw and open, which made the joy and tragedy we faced even more intense.

A little girl who pulled a pot of soup off the stove onto herself screams as the nurse and I clean and dress her horrible burns. A newborn cries vigorously after I give him oxygen and coax him into life. A little boy with very bad croup lies quietly in a mist tent, struggling to breathe. In the middle of a very long night at the intensive care unit, we realize that a baby boy suffering from a serious infection is going to live. A parent brings a little girl to the emergency room because of frequent headaches, only to be told that she has a brain tumor. A toddler, weak with a mysterious illness, laughs as she plays with my penlight. I close my eyes now and see those moments as clearly as if I were there again.

With the passage of time we gained knowledge and skills; with the passage of time we became comfortable and confident as doctors. At the end of three years we could continue up the medical hierarchy by doing a fellowship in a pediatric subspecialty, or we could go out and be general pediatricians, which is what I have done.

All of us going through medical training finish with a similar fund of knowledge. We know the causes of chest pain, which antibiotics to use for common infections, how to draw blood and interpret an X ray; we are well versed in most diseases and their treatments. However, we go about being doctors in very different ways. We have different styles of touching and talking to patients, different approaches to discussing difficult issues, different ways of sitting or standing when we discuss them. We have different priorities in the way we organize the workup of a symptom or plan of treatment. We have different expectations of our patients and, often, very different measures of success.

There are two components of medicine and its practice: the scientific and the emotional. The scientific is obvious and easily described; it is the tests, the drugs, the experiments, the biochemistry and pathology, and all the information that is readily accessible in textbooks. The emotional is less obvious and more difficult to describe; it has to do with the patient's and the doctor's feelings about illness and its treatment. It has a lot to do with relationships: the relationship between the doctor and the patient, between the patient and his family and friends, between the patient and his culture. The scientific and emotional components of medicine are often inseparable, each influencing and becoming part of the other.

There is a curriculum to teach the scientific component of medicine, one that is more or less standard throughout medical schools and residency programs. There is, however, no standard curriculum to teach the emotional component of medicine. It is recognized as important and discussed in varying depth at various times in medical training, but it is not easily taught; it is subtle and elusive and hard to explain.

We go about being doctors in different ways because of the differences in the way we practice the emotional component of medicine. Some of what we do we learned as part of growing up, long before we entered medical school, as we sorted out the kind of person we would be. We learn also from the example of doctors senior to us; we imitate the techniques and mannerisms of those we respect. We learn probably the most from the patients themselves, in times and places often unexpected, in moments that are etched into our minds or that slip quickly away, leaving only the lesson behind.

The circumstances under which doctors meet patients and their families are not ordinary; they are very personal, often stressful, and always vulnerable. Doctors meet patients and their families in the context of birth, death, pain, or joy, when keeping face is impossible or completely forgotten. Even when a patient goes to see a doctor for a routine checkup, doctors are allowed to ask personal questions and touch their bodies. Sometimes with eagerness, sometimes with reluctance, doctors are brought in and made witnesses to the bare moments, dramatic and mundane, that make up people's lives.

When my sister and I were children, my father would take us out simply to look and listen. We watched people in markets, puppies in pet stores, crabs at the beach; we watched sunsets silently while my father smoked one of his favorite cigars. We listened in on conversations and tried to figure out where people were from by their accents.

And always, we talked to people. We talked to the old ladies in the park, the man walking his dog, the mothers in the grocery store, the mailman. We knew all their names and where they lived and the latest news about their children. They probably thought my father eccentric, but he was so disarming, pleasant, and interested that they talked to us anyway.

I think that those times with my father had a lot to do with my decision to become a doctor. I grew to enjoy meeting people and entering into their lives in even a small way, and I thought that this was what doctors did. I thought they spent their days meeting people and helping them, helping them in ways that were special and powerful.

By the time I reached medical school I knew there was more to medicine than that, of course. I knew there was a tremendous amount of science I would need to learn. I knew being a doctor would be hard work. I knew I might face difficult ethical issues. I knew some patients die. I knew these things, but somehow my simple, shining image of a doctor as a powerful healer and friend prevailed, largely untouched. As I went through medical school and residency, many of the realities of medicine took me by surprise.

I didn't expect the study of medicine to be quite as overwhelming and disturbing as it sometimes was. I didn't expect that part of becoming a doctor would be learning a culture of jargon, habits, and beliefs. I didn't realize that I would be learning not only how to do something, but how to be someone, someone I didn't always want to be.

I wasn't prepared for how draining the practice of medicine would be. It was physically draining to be up all night and on my feet almost constantly, but it was even more draining emotionally. It was hard to be drawn into so many people's lives, to be part of their emotions as well as my own. It was hard to see people in pain, something I saw again and again every day. It was so hard to inflict pain, when I did something like draw blood or clean a burn, even though I was doing it to make someone better. It was especially hard to inflict pain on children. And I could never, ever, get used to watching someone die.

I didn't realize how ultimately limited medical science could be. I knew that we couldn't save everyone, but I didn't realize just how many we couldn't save or how many would have pain we couldn't ease. And I didn't realize how often illness and pain were caused by things like poverty, grief, neglect, loneliness— things that medical science could not touch. In so many situations what was required to help had nothing to do with drugs, surgery, or technology. The emotional component of medicine was incredibly pervasive and important, and it demanded more of me than I could ever have imagined.

My father taught me that every person has his or her story, and my life has become full of them. There have been people, conversations, relationships, and particular days or nights during my training that have affected me deeply and become intricately part of how I see the world.

The stories that I collected, that all of us going through medical training collect, are as much a part of that training as the textbooks, the lectures, the apprenticing, and everything else. They teach us the emotional component of medicine; they teach us how to be, and how we want to be, doctors. For me the stories are the best part of medicine. To know so many people and be witness to so much that is real and raw and deeply important is endlessly fascinating and completely worthwhile. The faces, the voices, and the moments are the enduring reasons I chose medicine and would never want to do anything else.

These are my stories.

LEARNING

HOW THE

HEART BEATS

HANDS

*T*he cadavers were laid out on tables, covered with white plastic sheets. We filed in quietly, leaving our backpacks in the hall, putting on lab coats and plastic gloves. We found our tables and busied ourselves with arranging our books and anatomical atlases and manuals, stealing glances at the shapeless white forms while making conversation with our partners, trying to act as though it didn't matter that there was a dead person in front of us.

"*R*espect," Professor Giardina had said to us earlier in his thick Italian accent, as we sat anxiously in the amphitheater awaiting our first dissection of the first-year Anatomy course. "You must always remember that these cadavers are not just objects, not just pieces of meat provided for your educational experience. These are people who lived lives and worked and played and loved just as you all do and will. These are people who chose to give you a very great gift. They gave you their bodies so that you might

1

learn, so that you might be better doctors. You may never give anyone such a great gift in your entire life."

He paused and pulled himself even straighter, staring out into the amphitheater as if at each one of us; I think we all squirmed. He raised his hand.

"So respect these people. Work carefully, and there will be no humor whatsoever at these people's expense. Treat each body as if it were your grandmother's body or your father's or yours there on that table. Now go. You should all have your assignments."

The smell of formaldehyde filled the lab rooms. It was sickening at first but became less noticeable over time. They were old rooms, with few windows and harsh lighting. The four of us stood there for what seemed like an eternity after we had arranged our books and equipment. I think Dan was first to make a move; he had taken Anatomy in college and didn't seem flustered at all. Once he took a corner of the sheet, the rest of us, startled, reached quickly to help.

Our cadaver was an old woman. I don't remember if we were told how old, but she seemed to be in her seventies. I know they didn't tell us what she died of, because I remember we kept looking for something, imagining ourselves medical examiners like the ones on television. Of course we didn't find anything or, if we did, we didn't recognize it. Her face and hands were covered with gauze bandages, as were those of all the cadavers. The instructors told us we were not to remove the gauze until we were told to do so. We obeyed; one did not disobey in Anatomy. It wasn't just wanting to get a good grade. It was awe.

We worked carefully for three hours, three mornings a week. Each day we were assigned a part of the body or organ system to dissect. We laid out our atlases and manuals and searched for the arteries, veins, nerves, muscles, and other structures we were asked to find. One person would read directions, another would find everything in the atlas, and the other two would do the actual dissecting with our brand-new scalpels, scissors, probes, and forceps. It was always harder to find things in the cadaver than in the atlas; the preserving process had turned most of the tissues grayish yellow. Veins looked like arteries, which looked like nerves, and the old woman's muscles were not as well defined as those in the illustrations in the atlas. The man in the atlas looked like a champion weight lifter.

It was fascinating work. We would study our atlases for hours at night and listen carefully to lectures, taking painstakingly complete notes, and then, in dissection, we would get to see everything laid out in a real human body. The intricacy and perfection of the design of the human body amazed me again and again. If the smartest people in the world were to sit down for months or years and try to design anything more perfect, I don't think they could do it. I don't think they could even have designed the human body as it is. The anatomy of each structure, from the microscopic parts of the kidney to the bones of the hand to the muscles of the legs, is exactly and elegantly suited to its function. We would carefully cut and probe the cadaver, able to see how it all worked together in a way the books alone couldn't show us. In the cadaver we could see the dimensions, the layers, the subtleties.

We worked steadily and seriously. We did some chatting, but not very much. The instructors would wander through the rooms, answering our questions and quizzing us. We usually finished late, quickly covering the cadaver with wet paper towels so it wouldn't dry out and then rushing out into the hallways, where people avoided walking near us because we stank of formaldehyde.

Dissecting the cadaver didn't bother me. I had been very worried that it would. The only other time I had ever seen a dead body was at my great-grandmother's wake when I was nine years old. I hadn't been able to imagine myself cutting into one, hovering over one, day after day.

But somehow, after that first lab, it wasn't hard. I guess I approached it as a task, as material to be learned, rather than as a dead body. I knew the cadaver was the body of a woman who had lived and breathed and loved and hated, but I didn't think of it that way. It made it easier to do the work if I didn't. I worried that not thinking of it that way meant I wasn't respecting her, but I figured that as long as my actions were respectful and I didn't make any jokes, I wasn't doing anything wrong. Well, at least nothing very wrong.

It didn't seem hard for any of my classmates, either; we took it in stride, or at least we appeared to. After all, this was a rite of initiation. This made us real medical students, that much closer to being doctors, and we felt comforted, more secure. We even carried ourselves differently; we walked with our heads held higher.

After each lab I would go back to my dorm room, take off my clothes, and put them in a plastic bag, which I closed up tightly so that the smell didn't take over the room. Then I would put on running clothes and sneakers and head for the Fens, the park near the medical school.

I didn't go far; there wasn't much time before the next class. I would run down Avenue Louis Pasteur, away from the medical school, and then turn right past the Isabella Stewart Gardner Museum and the Museum of Fine Arts. There were usually people out walking on the sidewalks or in the gardens of the Fens, and I liked to watch them as I ran. I would go up to the top of the Fens, where it meets Boylston Street near Kenmore Square, and then back down the other side past the Victory Gardens, where local people kept plots, past the playing fields, back to the medical school.

When people asked me why I went for my after-Anatomy

runs, I told them that the only way to get the smell out was to sweat it out, but it was more than that. I needed the running, the action itself, and I needed to get out and see people living ordinary lives. Running made it easier to go back the next time.

The day I remember best is the day we dissected the hands. I had wondered why the hands of all the cadavers were bandaged in gauze. I understood why the faces were covered; it would be upsetting to see the faces each day, and I had been relieved on the first day to find them wrapped in gauze. But the hands, the hands I couldn't understand.

We cut through the gauze and carefully peeled it away until the old woman's hands lay bare in front of us. I stood there and I stared at them, mesmerized.

My mind filled with images of hands. I thought of how I had stared at my own hands for hours as I practiced the piano, getting my finger positions perfect, straining to reach more than an octave in a Chopin piece, trying to keep them from getting tangled in a Bach two-part invention. I thought of my sister's hands on the same piano, younger, clumsier, somehow softer. I remembered the way my father held his pen when he drew pictures for us, the way his hands moved almost magically when he was making papier-mâché puppets or sculpting a figure out of clay. His fingers caressed and manipulated whatever it was he was working with and gave it life. I remembered how his hands felt when he picked us up: big, strong, capable. I thought of all the people I loved and realized I would probably know them all by their hands.

There is so much humanity in a pair of hands! Somehow I had not realized this, somehow I was not ready to see the old woman's small, thin hands laid out cold and dead in front of me. I wondered who would know her by her hands. Did she have a husband? Did she have children or grand-children whom she had held and caressed, who now thought of the sight and touch of her hands when she played with them or tucked them into bed?

They were thin hands, but they looked as though they had been strong. Not strong as if she had been a laborer, but strong as if she had used them often and well. I imagined them holding a needle and thread, sewing a hem or a sleeve. Maybe she knit; they looked like hands that would be quick and deft with knitting needles. Maybe she was a sculptress; I could see those hands gray with clay, working with a wet lump of it and shaping it into a figure. Maybe she played the piano; I wondered if she liked Chopin or Bach two-part inventions.

I remember the rest of that dissection well—at least I remember how the muscles and bones of the hands looked as we cut into and examined them—but I don't remember anything about what I did. I don't remember if I was cutting or reading instructions. I know that I wanted to leave, that I was upset and full of the knowledge that this cadaver was the body of a real person—but I was too embarrassed to say anything, too embarrassed to ask to leave. I searched the other faces in the room, trying to find some sign that someone was feeling the same way, but I could find nothing. Already we were learning to hide how we felt. I probably didn't show anything on my face, either.

I ran very fast after dissection that day, and I avoided the eyes of the people I saw, for I felt ashamed. Before then I had felt superior, privileged, privy to things the average person wasn't. But suddenly I felt ghoulish and strange, deeply disturbed by what I had spent so many hours doing. I had been cutting apart an old woman—not to take out a cancer or repair her in any way, but just to see how she was put together. I kept trying to tell myself that she was dead, that I wasn't hurting her, that this was a necessary part of medical school, but it didn't help. I ran harder and faster. I didn't think I could go back.

Of course I did go back. I had to go back if I was going to continue with medical school, if I was going to be a doctor, which was what I wanted more than anything. With time it got easier again, although it never was the same as before the hands. I tried again to concentrate on dissection as a task. I pushed aside the images, tried to find a place for them in my mind where they wouldn't bother me so much. Most of the time they stayed in that place. Sometimes they didn't.

The next time I went back I stood for a while at the side of the table where the old woman's body lay covered in its white sheet. Thank you, I said silently. I understand now about the gift.

MRS. ASGARIAN

*T*he subway train pulled into Maverick station. I stood up and held on to the railing until the train came to a full stop and the doors slid open in front of me. From behind me, three or four people walked purposefully out the doors, pushing me along with them. The station was big and open but dingy and a little dark. I made my way quickly to the wide stairs going up to the street.

The stairs led to an open square in East Boston with several buses parked in front of the subway entrance. It was January, and dirty snow lined the edges of the sidewalk. It was a cold, raw afternoon; people drew their coats around them as they walked quickly past me.

I pulled a crumpled piece of paper from my coat pocket, checked the bus route number I'd written there, and looked around for the bus. I found it, got on, and slid onto a seat near the front. I reread the rest of the directions on the piece of paper and put it back into my pocket.

It was my first home visit for "Plain Doctoring," a January course I was taking. January was separate from the rest of the academic year. Some people skipped it, went skiing or somewhere, and made up the credits later, but I had no place in particular I wanted to go. Various courses were offered, some more academically intense than others. I had chosen this one because it seemed interesting and not too demanding. After a long, difficult fall semester I wanted a break.

The course was run by three physicians at Massachusetts General Hospital. For one part of it, we read and discussed books by William Carlos Williams, Tillie Olsen, George Orwell, and other authors who wrote about the lives of people who were poor or ill or alone or about what it was like to work with them. For the other part, we visited people in their homes to talk with them about their feelings, their illnesses, their health care, their daily lives.

The bus wound its way through East Boston and across a bridge into Chelsea. I stared out the window. Many of the buildings and houses were old and in disrepair. Everything looked dirty, although it may just have been the January grime.

Up ahead I saw the apartment building I was looking for; it was exactly as Dr. Billings had described it. It was modern, or at least more modern than the surrounding buildings. Tall and boxy, made of what looked like gray cement, it was set back from the street and had a small parking lot. A wheelchair van and a laundry delivery truck were parked in front. I pulled the cord that ran above the bus window. The bus came to a stop at the corner, and I got out.

I went to the entrance. Dr. Billings had said it was an apartment building for senior citizens, for people who didn't need to be in a nursing home but needed help with laundry, grocery shopping, cleaning, rides to the doctor, and things like that. He made some house calls there; Mrs. Asgarian was one of his patients.

I was a little nervous. The last time I had spent time talking to someone who was old, besides my grandparents, was when I was in junior high school; I was part of a group of volunteers who visited a nursing home once a week. It was a good, clean nursing home, but still it smelled, a stale odor of urine, illness, and boredom. The people or clients or patients or whatever they were called sat on chairs or wheelchairs and stared at the television, the walls, one another, or nothing. Some were lost in worlds of their own, chattering unintelligibly; others were perfectly lucid and welcomed company. Although I liked listening to them, I never knew what to say back, and I would squirm uncomfortably on my chair. I wanted to help, I wanted to do something nice, but there was something about growing old that frightened me.

I went through a glass door into a small entranceway. On the wall was an intercom with rows of buttons, a name next to each. I ran my finger along the names, finally finding 7D: G. ASGARIAN. I pushed the button. Nothing happened. I pushed it again.

"Who's there?" came from the intercom. The voice was very faint.

"Mrs. Asgarian? It's Claire McCarthy, the medical student."

"Who?"

"The medical student. The one Dr. Billings told you would come. I called on Monday."

"Oh, yes. One moment."

The door buzzed and I opened it. The lobby was small, with tiled walls and orange indoor-outdoor carpeting. It smelled of disinfectant. A couple of metal folding chairs stood near the door. There was one elevator to the left; the up and down arrows were almost worn off the buttons. The elevator itself was tiny, and it creaked as it went up.

The hallway on the seventh floor was dark; one of the ceiling lights was out. The walls were an off white, the paint peeling in places, and the floor had the same orange carpeting as the lobby. It was very quiet, oddly quiet.

I knocked on the door marked 7D. I heard muffled footsteps.

"Who is it?"

"Claire McCarthy, Mrs. Asgarian. The medical student."

There was the sound of two bolts being pulled back and a chain undone. The door opened slightly and a small old woman peered out. She looked at me and then around me.

"It's just me, Mrs. Asgarian. There's nobody else here."

The door opened wider.

"Can't be too careful," she said, and motioned me inside.

She was only about five feet tall. She looked frail, but she moved with the slow precision of a dancer. Her wispy hair was dark gray and gathered neatly into a bun at the nape of her neck. Her skin was pale, almost transparent. She wore a cotton dress, too lightweight for the day's weather; it was a faded print, green with white flowers. Over it she wore a blue wool cardigan sweater that looked hand knit and was fraying at the elbows. On her feet were green quilted slippers; they looked new.

I was staring. She looked down at her clothes. "Is there something wrong?" she asked.

"No, of course not," I said, blushing. "I'm sorry."

She acknowledged my embarrassment with a nod and closed the door, putting the chain and the locks in place. She turned and looked at me. She had clear blue eyes, gentle eyes. I relaxed.

"Would you like to see my apartment? There isn't much to see, but Dr. Billings said you wanted to see how I live."

"Sure, I'd love to," I said, taking off my coat.

"You can leave your coat there," she said, pointing to a

hook on the wall by the door. She smiled. "I never use that hook. Can't reach it."

We were in a tiny entrance hallway. I followed her into the kitchen, which was immediately off to the right. It was small, almost cramped, with yellow walls and a yellow linoleum floor. It was drab, but clean; it smelled of the same disinfectant I'd smelled in the lobby. The appliances were small and old and the paint on the cabinets was cracking. Against the wall was a white metal table with two old chairs, one on either side. On the table was a round tray holding several medicine bottles and a bud vase with plastic flowers in it.

"I don't cook much anyway," she said.

Past the kitchen to the right was another short hallway, off which was the bedroom and the bathroom. I glanced quickly into them. The bathroom was tiny but clean, with flowered wallpaper. The bedroom was very dark (the shades were drawn tightly) and held a single bed and a dresser.

"And in here is my living room," she said, leading me back down the hallway.

It was the most pleasant room in the apartment. It was small but felt open and warm. There was plenty of light; the afternoon sun streamed in through the picture window that took up most of one wall. The carpeting was worn, and it was hard to tell what color it was—maybe blue, maybe gray. There was a slightly threadbare couch with a blue-and-yellow crocheted afghan draped over it, two other upholstered chairs, a coffee table, and an end table by one of the chairs. Several pictures hung on the walls. The room had an air of faded elegance.

"Please sit down," she said, pointing to the couch, and I did. She sat down on the wing chair across from me.

"I don't know what I am supposed to be telling you," she said. Her voice was soft, and she spoke slowly. "Dr. Billings didn't say very much. I'm supposed to tell you about my health problems?"

As it was my first visit and the instructions had been vague, I wasn't exactly sure what she was supposed to be telling me either. However, I didn't want to appear uncertain.

"I'd like to hear about your illnesses, yes, and your feelings about them and your doctors, if that's not too personal. I'd also like to hear about your life here."

She frowned. "I have heart failure, and there is something wrong with the way my heart beats—it shakes or something like that. They have some funny name for it—atra fib-something."

"Atrial fibrillation?"

"Yes, that's it. I have that, and I have arthritis. That's it."

I stifled the urge to take notes.

"I see," I said.

"Not very interesting, is it?"

"No, it's interesting." I just didn't know enough about atrial fibrillation, heart failure, or arthritis to ask follow-up questions. This was awkward. "And Dr. Billings is your doctor?"

"Yes."

"What do you think of him?"

"He's a very nice man."

"He is, isn't he."

We were quiet. I looked at my hands.

"Would you like to see my medicines?" she asked, standing up.

"I don't know very much yet about medicines. Please don't get up."

"No, I don't mind. It's good for me to get up. I'll bring them." She stood up slowly, supporting herself on the arms of the chair. When she was upright she stood very straight and then walked to the kitchen. She moved carefully, delicately.

I ran my fingers along the worn fabric of the couch. It was a thick fabric, with ornate medallions and bits of gold thread woven through. The arms of the couch were curved, with flowers carved into the wood. I leaned over to look more closely, admiring the intricately carved petals.

"It is beautiful, isn't it? It's the only good thing I have left. Here are my medicines." She handed me the round tray filled with medicines that had been on the kitchen table. "It was my mother's, and she loved it. I remember how she used to polish the wood every week. We were afraid to sit on it —we were afraid we'd spill something on it or put a hole in it. It still makes me nervous to sit on it, isn't that funny?" She looked at the couch with a distant smile for a moment, then looked back at me. "I've started some tea. You will join me, won't you?"

"Yes, thank you." She went back out to the kitchen. I picked up the pill containers. Digoxin, Coumadin, Lasix, Captopril, Halcion, Ibuprofen, Elavil, and Colace, they read. Digoxin and Ibuprofen I'd heard of; Digoxin was for heart problems and Ibuprofen for inflammation, probably for her arthritis. I thought Halcion might be a sleeping pill, but I wasn't sure. The rest I'd never heard of.

She came back into the room carrying a tray with a teapot and two cups and saucers. I jumped up and took it from her. "Please, let me," I said. I put it down on the coffee table.

"How do you take your tea?" she asked.

"Oh, plain is fine," I said.

She smiled. "That's how I take it, too. I'm sorry I don't have any cookies or pastry to offer you. I don't have money for extras these days."

"Oh, that's fine. May I?" She nodded, and I poured her a cup of tea. She sat down on the wing chair.

"What do you think of my medicines?"

"I'm afraid I haven't learned much yet about medicines," I said. "I'm only a first-year student. We don't take pharmacology until next semester."

"There are too many of them. I can never remember to take them all, and which ones I should take in the morning and which ones at night. It says on the bottles, but the writing is small, and it's hard for me to read sometimes, and then I forget what it said anyway."

"I'm sure Dr. Billings could help explain it all to you."

"Oh, he has. And the nurse who visits me twice a week helps me, too. But eight medicines is too many."

I looked down at my tea. What else was I supposed to ask her?

"Do you like this apartment?" I said.

"It's small, but it will do. Someone comes to clean, someone does the laundry, someone brings me groceries. Those things would be hard for me now. I am eighty-one, you know."

"How did you find this place?"

"My niece found it. She put me here. I don't blame her, really—she's got her own family, and she couldn't keep looking out for me."

"Does she live nearby?"

She leaned back on the chair. "No. She used to, but she moved away three or four years ago. She lives in Springfield now. Too far for her to come visit much. She used to visit a lot, with her children—it was nice. I liked watching them grow up. I couldn't leave here, though. This was the only place she could find that I could afford." She looked out the picture window. "It gets very quiet here. Nobody really comes to visit except the nurse and the doctor."

"What about the other people living here?"

"Oh, I know some of their names, but we don't visit. People here don't like to come out of their apartments. I knock sometimes when I know they're home, but a lot of the time they don't answer. Maybe they don't hear me. Maybe they're afraid—I get afraid sometimes when someone knocks at my door."

"What do you do during the day?"

"I read—I use a glass so I can see the words better, but it's getting harder. Sometimes I watch television, but there's not much I enjoy watching. I used to write lots of letters, but there aren't so many people to write to anymore. So many people I knew are dead now, you know."

She leaned back against the chair. The blue of her sweater reflected off her skin, and she looked almost ghostly.

"You could go out," I offered lamely.

"I could, I suppose," she said, "but I don't like to. It's hard for me to get around, and I don't know this town. I could get lost. Besides, this neighborhood isn't very safe."

She was right; it wasn't. I felt sorry that I had made her say these things. I was finding out what Dr. Billings wanted me to, probably, but it didn't seem fair to make her sad.

I put down my teacup and stood up. There were some old framed photographs on the wall by the window. I went over to look at them.

The one closer to the window was of a young man standing at the bottom of some steps in front of a brick building. He wore a suit and hat. One foot was on the bottom step, and his hands were in his pockets. His head was cocked slightly to one side, and there was something irrepressible about his expression. He looked as though he were about to tell a joke or tease the photographer.

"Who's this?" I asked.

"My husband," said Mrs. Asgarian.

"He was very handsome," I said. He was; he was tall, with dark hair, a long, angled face, and friendly dark eyes.

"Oh, no picture could show you how handsome he was," said Mrs. Asgarian. "The way he moved was handsome. The way he talked was handsome. Everything about him was handsome."

The other picture was a wedding picture, brown with age. It was a formal, posed picture of Mrs. Asgarian and her husband. His arm encircled her waist, holding her close to him. He wore a dark suit. She wore a simple, fitted white dress that almost reached the floor. The face was recognizable as hers, but just barely. Only her eyes, her nose, and the way she carried herself were the same. In the picture she was as beautiful as he was handsome, and looked just as irrepressible.

I turned to Mrs. Asgarian. The afternoon sun was growing dimmer, but it was in her eyes as she faced me. She held her hand up to block it and squinted. She seemed small and fragile on the big wing chair, and her hand shook as she held it up. I sat back down on the couch.

"How did you meet him?" I asked.

"I was working in a dress factory," she said. "It broke my father's heart that I had to do such work—he had come from Poland to make a better life, he said, and now his children were working. But we had no choice. We had a big family, and there wasn't enough money, so my sister and I went to work, and the dress factory was all we could find. It was bad work. They paid us very little, and we worked long, long days, sewing until our fingers were very sore."

She looked at her hands, rubbing her fingertips.

"Adam—that is my husband—he was a, what would you say, an organizer. He worked for the union. He would wait outside and talk to us when we came in and when we left. It made the owners very angry. We were afraid to talk to him, because we thought we would lose our jobs. But there was something about him—I had to talk to him. So one day I said hello to him."

"Just hello?"

She laughed at me. "Not only was that enough for me to lose my job, it was very improper for a young lady to approach a young man. Times were very different then."

"What did he say?"

"He tipped his hat and said hello to me, too. And he smiled. What a smile! I think I fell in love that moment." Her eyes looked off toward the pictures on the wall.

"So then what happened?"

"Nothing, for a long time. We said hello outside the factory, but he did not come to call. It would have been improper, without an introduction. We would just say hello, and we would smile. I tried to do it so that nobody would see. Then one day he came up to me as I was leaving the factory. Later he told me that he had fallen in love with me, too, and that he felt like he had to speak to me. He came up to me, and he touched my arm, only for a tiny moment, and he said, 'My name is Adam Asgarian. Please, would you tell me your name?' 'Grace,' I said. 'Grace Vlacek.'

"And he stood there, and his eyes were so full, and I will never forget what he said. 'What a perfect name for you,' he said. 'I have never seen anyone more full of grace than you.'"

I could imagine what he would have looked like as he said that. I could almost see him standing there on the street with his eyes so full.

"We were married a few months later. My family was very upset, even though he was Jewish. They did not like how we met, they didn't think our courtship was proper. They could not understand how we felt, how we knew we had to be married. They did not come to the wedding. We had, what do you call it—a civil ceremony. It made me sad not to have a canopy, not to have my family, but I had Adam, and that was all that mattered to me."

I had moved to the edge of the couch, my hands clasped in my lap. "Where did you live?"

"We had an apartment in Roxbury—it was very different then from the way it is now. There were a lot of Jewish people there, it was a nice community."

"Did your husband keep working for the union?"

"For a while, yes. But he was taking law classes, and as soon as he got his degree he opened up a small practice. I helped him out in the office. We were always together." Her eyes stayed on the picture, as if she were talking to him.

"I worked as his secretary, and he taught me law, too—I loved to learn. We would work all day together, and then we would eat lovely meals—we didn't have much money, but I always tried to make nice meals. And then we would read books together or talk late into the night about everything."

"Did you have any children?"

"No," she said. "We never did. I don't know why. But Adam, he always said it didn't matter, that maybe it was better that we didn't have any children. He said he loved me so much, he didn't know if he'd ever be able to share me with children. We had a lovely life, though. I was never sad that we didn't have children until after he died. Then I wished we'd had children so that there might be some part of him still living."

"When did he die?" I asked hesitantly.

She sighed, shifted on her chair. "A long, long time ago," she said. "Nineteen fifty-one. January nineteenth. He was hit by a truck. The police came to tell me. It was cold, and it was raining, and they came to the door, and they told me."

The afternoon sun was almost gone. The room was grow-

ing dark, and I could not see her face very well in the shadow
of the chair.

"Nothing was the same after he was gone," she said. Her
voice was so soft, I could barely hear it. "I found work as a
secretary, and I read lots of books and had many friends,
but nothing was ever the same."

"I'm sorry," I said.

She was quiet. There was no sound except the sound of
an occasional car going by outside, but the silence was very
full.

"Don't be sorry," she said finally. "I'm not sorry. I had
Adam, and I could never ask anything more of life. But the
days, the days are long."

I looked at her, and I thought, I could never be her doctor. I couldn't hear these stories, I couldn't know these things
about her and be her doctor, too. How did doctors do it?
Was it better not to find out things about people? I wouldn't
be able to lecture her about taking her medicines. I wouldn't
be able to ask her to take off her clothes and then examine
her, see her naked and touch her and ask her to breathe
deeply while I listened to her lungs. I could never have
enough distance; it would feel like a violation.

And, I realized as I looked at the old woman wrapped in
the shadows, it would be too hard to know that I could do
nothing to treat the real disease of her heart.

DOG LAB

When I finished college and started medical school, the learning changed fundamentally. Whereas in college I had been learning mostly for learning's sake, learning in order to know something, in medical school I was learning in order to *do* something, do the thing I wanted to do with my life. It was exhilarating and at the same time a little scary. My study now carried responsibility.

The most important course in the first year besides Anatomy was Physiology, the study of the functions and processes of the human body. It was the most fascinating subject I had ever studied. I found the intricacies of the way the body works endlessly intriguing and ingenious: the way the nervous system is designed to differentiate a sharp touch from a soft one; the way muscles move and work together to throw a ball; the wisdom of the kidneys, which filter the blood and let pass out only waste products and extra fluid, keeping everything else carefully within. It was magical to me that each organ and system worked so beautifully and in perfect concert with the rest of the body.

The importance of Physiology didn't lie just in the fact that it was fascinating, however. The other courses I was taking that semester, like Histology and Biochemistry, were fascinating, too. But because Physiology was the study of how the body actually works, it seemed the most pertinent to becoming a physician. The other courses were more abstract. Physiology was practical, and I felt that my ability to master Physiology would be a measure of my ability to be a doctor.

When the second-year students talked about Physiology, they always mentioned "dog lab." They mentioned it briefly but significantly, sharing knowing looks. I gathered that it involved cutting dogs open and that it was controversial, but that was all I knew. I didn't pursue it, I didn't ask questions. That fall I was living day to day, lecture to lecture, test to test. My life was organized around putting as much information into my brain as possible, and I didn't pay much attention to anything else.

I would get up around six, make coffee, and eat my bowl of cereal while I sat at my desk. There was nowhere else to sit in my dormitory room, and if I was going to sit at my desk, I figured I might as well study, so I always studied as I ate. I had a small refrigerator and a hot plate so that I could fix myself meals. After breakfast it was off to a morning of lectures, back to the room at lunchtime for a yogurt or soup and more studying, then afternoon lectures and labs. Before dinner I usually went for a run or a swim; although it was necessary for my sanity and my health, I always felt guilty that I wasn't studying instead. I ate dinner at my desk or with other medical students at the cafeteria in Beth Israel Hospital. We sat among the doctors, staff, and patients, eat-ing our food quickly. Although we would try to talk about movies, current affairs, or other "nonmedical" topics, sooner or later we usually ended up talking about medicine; it was fast becoming our whole life. After dinner it was off to the eerie quiet of the library, where I sat surrounded by my textbooks and notes until I got tired or frustrated, which was usually around ten-thirty. Then I'd go back to the dorm, maybe chat with the other students on my floor, maybe watch television, probably study some more, and then fall asleep so that I could start the routine all over again the next morning.

My life had never been so consuming. Sometimes I felt like a true student in the best sense of the word, wonderfully absorbed in learning; other times I felt like an automaton. I was probably a combination of the two. It bothered me sometimes that this process of teaching me to take care of people was making me live a very study-centered, self-centered life. However, it didn't seem as though I had a choice.

One day at the beginning of a physiology lecture the instructor announced that we would be having a laboratory exercise to study the cardiovascular system, and that dogs would be used. The room was quickly quiet; this was the infamous "dog lab." The point of the exercise, he explained, was to study the heart and blood vessels in vivo, to learn the effects of different conditions and chemicals by seeing them rather than just by reading about them. The dogs would be sedated and the changes in their heart rates, respiratory rates, and blood pressure would be monitored with each experiment. As the last part of the exercise the sleeping dogs' chests would be cut open so we could actually watch the hearts and lungs in action, and then the dogs would be killed, humanely. We would be divided up into teams of four, and each team would work with a teaching assistant. Because so many teaching assistants were required, the class would be divided in half, and the lab would be held on two days.

The amphitheater buzzed.

The lab was optional, the instructor told us. We would not be marked off in any way if we chose not to attend. He leaned against the side of the podium and said that the way he saw it there was a spectrum of morality when it came to animal experimentation. The spectrum, he said, went from mice or rats to species like horses or apes, and we had to decide at which species we would draw our lines. He hoped, though, that we would choose to attend. It was an excellent learning opportunity, and he thought we ought to take advantage of it. Then he walked behind the podium and started the day's lecture.

It was all anyone could talk about: should we do dog lab or shouldn't we? We discussed it endlessly.

There were two main camps. One was the "excellent learning opportunity" camp, which insisted that dog lab was the kind of science we came to medical school to do and that learning about the cardiovascular system on a living animal would make it more understandable and would therefore make us better doctors.

Countering them was the "importance of a life" camp. The extreme members of this camp insisted that it was always wrong to murder an animal for experimentation. The more moderate members argued that perhaps animal experimentation was useful in certain kinds of medical research, but that dog lab was purely an exercise for our education and didn't warrant the killing of a dog. We could learn the material in other ways, they said.

On and on the arguments went, with people saying the same things over and over again in every conceivable way. There was something very important about this decision.

Maybe it was because we were just beginning to figure out how to define ourselves as physicians—were we scientists, eager for knowledge, or were we defenders of life? The dog lab seemed to pit one against the other. Maybe it was because we thought that our lives as physicians were going to be filled with ethical decisions, and this was our first since entering medical school. It was very important that we do the right thing, but the right thing seemed variable and unclear.

I was quiet during these discussions. I didn't want to kill a dog, but I certainly wanted to take advantage of every learning opportunity offered me. And despite the fact that the course instructor had said our grades wouldn't be affected if we didn't attend the lab, I wasn't sure I believed him, and I didn't want to take any chances. Even if he didn't incorporate the lab report into our grades, I was worried that there would be some reference to it in the final exam, some sneaky way that he would bring it up. Doing well had become so important that I was afraid to trust anyone; doing well had become more important than anything.

I found myself waiting to see what other people would decide. I was ashamed not to be taking a stand, but I was stuck in a way I'd never been before. I didn't like the idea of doing the lab; it felt wrong. Yet for some reason I was embarrassed that I felt that way, and the lab seemed so important. The more I thought about it, the more confused I became.

Although initially the students had appeared divided more or less evenly between the camps, as the lab day drew nearer the majority chose to participate. The discussions didn't stop, but they were fewer and quieter. The issue seemed to become more private.

I was assigned to the second lab day. My indecision was becoming a decision since I hadn't crossed my name off the list. I can still change my mind, I told myself. I'm not on a team yet, nobody's counting on me to show up. One of my classmates asked me to join his group. I hedged.

The day before group lists had to be handed in, the course instructor made an announcement. It was brief and almost offhand: he said that if any of us wished to help anesthetize the dogs for the lab, we were welcome to do so. He told us where to go and when to be there for each lab day. I wrote the information down.

Somehow, this was what I needed. I made my decision. I would do the lab, but I would go help anesthetize the dogs first.

Helping with the anesthesia, I thought, would be taking full responsibility for what I was doing, something that was very important to me. I was going to *face* what I was doing, see the dogs awake with their tails wagging instead of meeting them asleep and sort of pretending they weren't real. I also thought it might make me feel better to know that the dogs were treated well as they were anesthetized and to be there, helping to do it gently. Maybe in part I thought of it as my penance.

*T*he day of the first lab came. Around five o'clock I went down to the Friday afternoon "happy hour" in the dormitory living room to talk to the students as they came back. They came back singly or in pairs, quiet, looking dazed. They threw down their coats and backpacks and made their way to the beer and soda without talking to anyone. Some, once they had a cup in their hands, seemed to relax and join in conversations; others took their cups and sat alone on the couches. They all looked tired, worn out.

"Well?" I asked several of them. "What was it like?"

Most shrugged and said little. A few said that it was in-teresting and that they'd learned a lot, but they said it without any enthusiasm. Every one of them said it was hard. I thought I heard someone say that their dog had turned out to be pregnant. Nobody seemed happy.

The morning of my lab was gray and dreary. I overslept, which I hardly ever do. I got dressed quickly and went across the street to the back entrance of the lab building. It was quiet and still and a little dark. The streets were empty except for an occasional cab. I found the open door and went in.

There was only one other student waiting there, a blond-haired woman named Elise. I didn't know her well. We had friends in common, but we'd never really talked. She was sweet and soft-spoken; she wore old jeans and plaid flannel shirts and hung out with the activist crowd. She had always intimidated me. I felt as though I weren't political enough when I was around her. I was actually a little surprised that she was doing the lab at all, as many of her friends had chosen not to.

We greeted each other awkwardly, nodding hello and taking our places leaning against the wall. Within a few minutes one of the teaching assistants came in, said good morning, pulled out some keys, and let us into a room down the hall. Two more teaching assistants followed shortly.

The teaching assistants let the dogs out of cages, and they ran around the room. They were small dogs; I think they were beagles. They seemed happy to be out of their cages, and one of them, white with brown spots, came over to me with his tail wagging. I leaned over to pet him, and he licked my hand, looking up at me eagerly. I stood up again quickly.

The teaching assistant who had let us in, a short man with tousled brown hair and thick glasses, explained that the dogs were to be given intramuscular injections of a sedative that would put them to sleep. During the lab they would be given additional doses intravenously as well as other medications to stop them from feeling pain. We could help, he said, by holding the dogs while they got their injections. Elise and I nodded.

So we held the dogs, and they got their injections. After a few minutes they started to stumble, and we helped them to the floor. I remember that Elise petted one of the dogs as he fell asleep and that she cried. I didn't cry, but I wanted to.

When we were finished, I went back to my room. I sat at my desk, drank my coffee, and read over the lab instructions again. I kept thinking about the dogs running around, about the little white one with the brown spots, and I felt sick. I stared at the instructions without really reading them, looking at my watch every couple of minutes. At five minutes before eight I picked up the papers, put them in my backpack with my books, and left.

The lab was held in a big open room with white walls and lots of windows. The dogs were laid out on separate tables lined up across the room; they were on their backs, tied down. They were all asleep, but some of them moved slightly, and it chilled me.

We walked in slowly and solemnly, putting our coats and backpacks on the rack along the wall and going over to our assigned tables. I started to look for the dog who had licked my hand, but I stopped myself. I didn't want to know where he was.

Our dog was brown and black, with soft floppy ears. His eyes were shut. He looked familiar. We took our places, two on each side of the table, laid out our lab manuals, and began.

The lab took all day. We cut through the dog's skin to find an artery and vein, into which we placed catheters. We injected different drugs and chemicals and watched what happened to the dog's heart rate and blood pressure, carefully recording the results. At the end of the day, when we were done with the experiments, we cut open the dog's chest. We cut through his sternum and pulled open his rib cage. His heart and lungs lay in front of us. The heart was a fist-size muscle that squeezed itself as it beat, pushing blood out. The lungs were white and solid and glistening under the pleura that covered them. The instructor pointed out different blood vessels, like the aorta and the superior vena cava. He showed us the stellate ganglion, which really did look like a star. I think we used the electrical paddles of a defibrillator and shocked the dog's heart into ventricular fibrillation, watching it shiver like Jell-O in front of us. I think that's how we killed them—or maybe it was with a lethal dose of one of the drugs. I'm not sure. It's something I guess I don't want to remember.

Dan was the anesthesiologist, the person assigned to making sure that the dog stayed asleep throughout the entire procedure. Every once in a while Dan would get caught up in the experiment and the dog would start to stir. I would nudge Dan, and he would quickly give more medication. The dog never actually woke up, but every time he moved even the slightest bit, every time I had to think about him being a real dog who was never going to wag his tail or lick anyone's hand again because of us, I got so upset that I couldn't concentrate. In fact, I had trouble concentrating on the lab in general. I kept staring at the dog.

As soon as we were finished, or maybe a couple of minutes before, I left. I grabbed my coat and backpack and ran down the stairs out into the dusk of the late afternoon. It was drizzling, and the medical school looked brown and gray. I walked quickly toward the street.

I was disappointed in the lab and disappointed in myself

for doing it. I knew now that doing the lab was wrong. Maybe not wrong for everyone—it was clearly a complicated and individual choice—but wrong for me. The knowledge I had gained wasn't worth the life of a dog to me. I felt very sad.

The drizzle was becoming rain. I slowed down; even though it was cold, the rain felt good. A couple of people walking past me put up their umbrellas. I let the rain fall on me. I wanted to get wet.

From the moment you enter the field of medicine as a medical student, you have an awareness that you have entered something bigger and more important than you are. Doctors are different from other people, we are told implicitly, if not explicitly. Medicine is a way of life, with its own values and guidelines for daily living. They aren't bad values; they include things like the importance of hard work, the pursuit of knowledge, and the preservation of life—at least human life. There's room for individuality and variation, but that's something I realized later, much later. When I started medical school I felt that not only did I have to learn information and skills, I had to become a certain kind of person, too. It was very important to me to learn to do the thing that a doctor would do in a given situation. Since the course instructor, who represented Harvard Medical School to me, had recommended that we do the lab, I figured that a doctor would do it. That wasn't the only reason I went ahead with the lab, but it was a big reason.

The rain started to come down harder and felt less pleasant. I walked more quickly, across Longwood Avenue into Vanderbilt Hall. I could hear familiar voices coming from the living room, but I didn't feel like talking to anyone. I ducked into the stairwell.

I got to my room, locked the door behind me, took off my coat, and lay down on my bed. The rain beat against my window. It was the time I usually went running, but the thought of going back out in the rain didn't appeal to me at all. I was suddenly very tired.

As I lay there I thought about the course instructor's discussion of the spectrum of morality and drawing lines. Maybe it's not a matter of deciding which animals I feel comfortable killing, I thought. Maybe it's about drawing different kinds of lines: drawing the lines to define how much of myself I will allow to change. I was proud of being a true student, even if it did mean becoming a little like an automaton. But I still needed to be the person I was before; I needed to be able to make some decisions without worrying about what a doctor would do.

I got up off the bed, opened a can of soup, and put it in a pan on the hot plate to warm. I got some bread and cheese out of the refrigerator, sat down at my desk, and opened my Biochemistry text.

Suddenly I stopped. I closed the text, reached over, and turned on the television, which sat on a little plastic table near the desk. There would be time to study later. I was going to watch television, read a newspaper, and call some friends I hadn't called since starting medical school. It was time to make some changes, some changes back.

THE LAYING
ON OF
HANDS

Dr. Hilder stood in front of us and, in a voice that we sometimes had to strain to hear, welcomed us to New England Deaconess Hospital and to Introduction to Clinical Medicine. I sat with Peter, Rebecca, and the fifteen or so other second-year students, feeling self-conscious and wonderful in the white coat I had just been given by an old woman in the hospital laundry.

"Thirty-six?" she said as I handed her the voucher. "Here." She threw it on the counter, and it slipped toward the floor. I grabbed it quickly. This is my first white coat, I thought. It can't fall on the floor.

"In this course," said Dr. Hilder, "we will teach you the skills you need to enter your clinical rotations. We will teach you how to take a history, how to present on rounds, and, of course, how to do a physical exam."

"This," Peter said later as we ate lunch in the hospital cafeteria, "is when we learn the laying on of hands."

*T*here was a clear division between the students in the first two years of Harvard Medical School and those in the second two: those in the first two years didn't know how to do a physical exam, and those in the second two did. As first- and second-year students, we were very aware of this difference and looked at the third- and fourth-year students with some awe when we saw them with their white coats and stethoscopes on the way to one of the hospitals. Their world seemed so much more interesting and exciting, and it was hard not to be jealous, hard not to be anxious to get to where they were.

Introduction to Clinical Medicine, or ICM, as we called it, was our passage. It was a mandatory course given at the end of the second year that met three days a week. The class was divided up among the hospitals associated with Harvard. We were given a list of the medical instruments we would need, and off we went to the medical supply store. We were like children in a toy store, picking out our first stethoscopes, choosing which ophthalmoscope kit we wanted, looking at the different kinds of reflex hammers. I bought more than I needed to buy, wanting to be prepared for anything. I went back to my dorm room and laid everything out on my bed, marveling at these wonderful things I now owned.

We squirmed through the lectures on taking a medical history. Reflexively we took good notes, laborious notes, on questions we were supposed to ask the patients, the order in which we were to ask them, and the way in which we were to write down responses in our admission notes. We listened carefully but not patiently, waiting for the lecture to be over so we could learn another part of the physical exam.

We started with the head. First one of the specialists from the Deaconess lectured to us, showing slides on techniques and what to look for, and then he demonstrated what to do, using one of us as a model. Afterward we paired up and practiced on each other; Rebecca was my partner. We took out our brand-new otoscopes and ophthalmoscopes, awkwardly trying to figure out how to put them together and then how to use them.

Once I'd put mine together and found out how to look through it, I was riveted. I had never seen an eardrum before, and it wasn't what I expected. It looked like waxed paper, with a little triangle of light reflecting back, and if I looked closely, I could see the tiny bones of the middle ear behind the waxed-paper membrane. And the retina—it was amazing! All those tiny blood vessels weaving intricately across its surface and coming together on the bright, round optic disc. I watched Rebecca's pupils get smaller as I shined light on them, and change as I had her look at something near, then far. It was just like the textbooks said it would be.

Over the ensuing days we learned to use our fingers to search for swollen glands or an enlarged thyroid in the neck. Our instructors taught us to listen carefully with our stethoscopes for pneumonia, wheezing, or other sounds in the lungs. We learned how to listen to each heart sound, how to listen for clicks and murmurs, how to know where they were in the cardiac cycle, and how to describe them. We learned how to feel abdomens, looking for a big liver or spleen or a mass that shouldn't be there. We learned how to examine breasts and genitals. We learned to look at hands and feet and arms and legs and spines, how to look for skin problems, how to do a neurological examination. The human body was being made accessible to us.

At lunchtime we talked incessantly about what we were learning. There were six or so of us who usually ate together in the big, bright, crowded cafeteria. There were a few patients and visitors who ate there, but mostly it was staff: administration, support staff, nurses, and doctors. I liked looking at the doctors, whenever I could do so without being caught. Their white coats were more crumpled and looked more comfortable on them than ours did on us. The pockets of their coats were filled with just the right number of useful things, like a pen, a penlight, and some index cards. We'd filled our pockets with so much stuff, "just in case," that our coats sagged. I liked to watch the easy way the doctors sat, the easy way they got up when they were done and sauntered out. I liked to listen in on conversations, especially when they were talking about work or patients. I liked hearing the words and phrases they used. Sometimes it was like listening to a foreign language.

Except for the examinations of the breasts and genitals, which we practiced on willing healthy people recruited by Dr. Hilder, we continued to practice on each other. Our enthusiasm and curiosity helped allay some of the embarrassment, but it was awkward. Touching is, or at least can be, so personal. It can be so significant to reach over and touch someone's sleeve, so tremendously difficult to take someone's hand, and we were doing much more than that to each other and later to people we'd never met before. We were getting close, so close in some parts of the examination that they could feel our breath on their skin.

Someone once brought up the awkwardness with one of the instructors, who brushed it off. "You have to learn to do this to be doctors," he said, and that was the end of it. We didn't talk about it anymore, and if we were embarrassed, we tried not to show it.

Once we had practiced part of the examination on each other, we would be taken in small groups to see patients who had "interesting physical findings." We would take turns listening to heart murmurs, feeling enlarged livers, or whatever else the instructors could find for us among the patients in the hospital. The patients were generally gracious and pleasant. They allowed us to touch them and listen to them with our stethoscopes and look at parts of their bodies usually kept carefully covered. It was wonderful. Since we were healthy, when we examined each other we were mostly just going through the motions; there wasn't much to find. With the patients, we went through the motions—and found things. We tried to act professional and reserved, but I'm sure our excitement was obvious.

I had been thinking that maybe one of the reasons patients didn't mind doctors touching them was that doctors touched with confidence and purpose. We certainly didn't have confidence, and there wasn't much purpose to what we were doing, yet the patients didn't seem to mind. It was something else, something that had to do with our white coats or our hospital identification badges. When we put them on and draped our stethoscopes around our necks, we became people who were part of the medical profession; we became people who were allowed to touch. Not every patient was completely comfortable with us, but our investigations were always allowed. It made me feel powerful in a way I hadn't quite expected.

As the next step in our training, we were sent off on our own to do histories and physicals on agreeable patients recruited by the instructors. It was nice to be on my own, away from the embarrassingly obvious group of students, but I missed the guidance of having others to watch. I sat on chairs in corners of hospital rooms, asking long lists of questions because I wasn't sure what was important to ask, and then I would do the physical exam. I was still learning on which side to stand and which hand to use to hold the otoscope or to feel patients' abdomens, still trying to remember all the things I was supposed to look at and in which order, and at the same time trying to keep in my head all the things I had found. (What was that blood pressure again? Which side of his mouth drooped?) I was understandably tense. I hoped the patients didn't notice, but some of them must have.

We were paired up with doctors who had volunteered to be instructors in the course. They went over our physical exams with us and taught us how to write admission notes. They taught us, too, how to "present" patients. Presenting is something that is done on rounds, usually on your feet, preferably from memory or with minimal help from notes. The idea is to succinctly (in no more than seven minutes) tell the rest of the doctors on the team about the patient's problems, his or her medical history, pertinent family and social history, physical exam, laboratory values, and radiologic studies. To do it properly you must stand straight, speak audibly and with authority, and use telegraphic sentences filled with the kinds of medical phrases and abbreviations I had overheard in the cafeteria.

I practiced and practiced, and slowly something began to emerge. The language became easier, the sentence structure more natural, and I began to understand what the doctors in the cafeteria were saying. During the physical exams my fingers became more adept and sensitive. They learned to feel for big lumps and tiny things, for textures and asymmetries. They became confident and organized, moving in a predictable way down a neck, across an abdomen, around a joint. I learned how to listen intently through my stethoscope, to pick up little sounds: a faint crackle in the lungs signifying the presence of fluid, the blowing of a soft heart murmur. I learned to watch and to look carefully, to notice small rashes or that someone dragged his foot slightly when he walked.

The touching became easier, too. I worked at draining the personal from my fingertips, at concentrating on what I was looking and feeling for rather than on the patient. It was a matter of being there but not being there, of being present as physician, but not as peer or friend. That's not to say I wasn't friendly or that later I was never friends with my patients; it's just that doing physical exams requires some distance, especially at the beginning.

The white coat, the stethoscope, and the language of medicine helped. The culture of medicine set us apart from the patients.

We started to feel as if we belonged among the people in the cafeteria. Our pockets were still too full, but it bothered us less. We sat more comfortably on our chairs, leaning back, and we used medical jargon and phraseology whenever we could.

I had so many daydreams as I walked home at the end of the day. I would imagine myself making difficult diagnoses just based on the history and the findings of my thorough, perfectly done physical exams. My touch would be so gentle, so supportive, that even the sickest of patients would feel a little healed when I left the room.

One day toward the end of the course I was sent to take a history from and examine a patient named Meredith Vane. Mrs. Vane, my instructor told me, was a fifty-one-year-old woman suffering from amyloidosis. Amyloidosis is one of those rare and scientifically interesting diseases that we seemed to learn a lot about in medical school. It is a disease in which a protein called amyloid is deposited in organs and tissues all over the body; it collects in the heart, the kidneys, the liver, the lungs, the skin— everywhere. As it collects, it interferes with the function of the organ or tissue. Sometimes the amyloid is deposited as part of an infection or illness; sometimes it is there, inexplicably, by itself. It varies in extent and severity, but we had been taught that in general it was slowly progressive and incurable. In Pathology we'd looked under the microscope at specimens of a kidney filled with amyloid. The normal architecture was distorted with a pink, glassy substance. It was sort of pretty, the way it sparkled under the light. I was very interested to meet someone who actually had the disease.

Meredith Vane was propped up in bed on several pillows. The curtains were drawn back, and the room was filled with sunshine. Two of the walls were nearly covered with get-well cards, and there was a vase of yellow flowers on the metal dresser. Instead of a hospital blanket, her bed was covered with a green-and-blue patchwork quilt.

I introduced myself.

"Oh, yes," she said, "the medical student who's here to give me an extra physical."

I opened my mouth to say something, although I wasn't sure what to say.

"Oh, don't worry," she said with a smile. "An extra physical never hurt anyone. What did you say your name was? Claire?"

I nodded.

"You must call me Meredith. I don't like to be called Mrs. Vane—makes me sound like my mother-in-law, and I sure don't want that." She chuckled, and I laughed, too.

She was a large woman with a round face. It was hard to tell how heavy she was because she was wearing a big flannel nightgown, and most of her was covered by the quilt. She had wonderful hair; it was long and wavy and auburn, with a few streaks of gray that made it all the more interesting. Her face was pale and a little puffy, but she looked younger than fifty-one. She had broad, handsome features and deep green eyes.

I sat on the chair next to the bed, pulled out my clipboard, and dug in my pockets for a pen.

Meredith watched me. "How much stuff do you have in those pockets, anyway?"

I blushed. "It's just stuff I need." I found a pen.

"You need all that? You poor thing. You remind me of a little boy with too many things in his pockets. Any worms in there?"

"No," I said. "I left them at home today."

She grinned. "I like you," she said. "So what do you want to do to me?"

"Actually, if it's okay, I'd like to ask some questions first."

She groaned. "Oh, they didn't tell me this. Couldn't you just find out what you need from my chart? They have taught you about charts, haven't they?"

"It'd be better if I could get it from you," I said.

"Oh, but it's such a boring story," she said. "I went to my doctor because I was having trouble breathing whenever I walked even a short distance, and he said I had heart failure. Then it turned out that there was protein in my urine. It took almost a year before they figured out what was going on with me—apparently this amyloidosis thing is pretty rare. That was almost four years ago. Things haven't exactly been going well since."

She reached over and opened the drawer of the bedside table and pulled out a manila envelope.

"These just came today. I've been dying to show them to somebody," she said, opening the envelope and taking out some pictures. "They are of my older daughter at her wedding in February. See, there's Emily. That's her husband, Jim. Nice guy. My daughter did well."

I tried to ask her specific questions about her symptoms and what she meant by "Things haven't exactly been going well since," but it was hard to get answers from her. She wanted to show me the wedding pictures, and then she pulled out pictures of her other daughter for me to see.

"This is Andrea. You remind me a little of her—she's tall, too, and see, you two have similar faces."

I didn't see the resemblance, but I nodded.

"She's twenty-three, just turned a couple of months ago —these pictures are from a birthday party they had for her out in L.A.—that's where she lives. She just got engaged. They're not getting married until next June, though. Gives me plenty of time to plan the wedding!"

I looked at all the pictures, and we talked about planning weddings. Her eyes sparkled as she talked about her daughters. She told me that before she got sick she used to be a photographer, and she pulled her portfolio out of the bottom drawer of the dresser for me to look at. It was filled with black-and-white pictures of children and animals and seascapes and touching little moments, like one of an old man kissing his wife on a park bench. They were great pictures—sensitive, interesting, moments captured rather than posed.

I looked at my watch. I had to meet with my instructor in an hour, and I needed to have finished everything and written something up by then.

She saw me looking. "Okay, okay, you want your history. Well, you can get the details from my chart, but since I was diagnosed my heart failure and my kidneys have been getting worse, despite a ton of medications that they keep changing all the time. They've been talking about doing dialysis, but I guess my kidneys aren't quite that bad yet. I've had problems with my intestines, too, but those aren't so bad. My breathing is getting harder, and they think I might have some amyloid in my lungs, but they're not sure. I've been here for about three weeks now. I couldn't get around at all at home, so they're trying yet another experimental therapy.

My doctor is really optimistic about this one. Says he's sure it's going to help. That's all you need to know, right?"

It wasn't, of course. I was supposed to get detailed information about her past medical history, including dates. I was supposed to get a list of her medications and their dosages. I was supposed to find out about illnesses among people in her family. I was supposed to go through a complete review of systems, asking about every possible symptom from head to toe.

I looked at her. She still had the portfolio on her lap, and the other pictures were scattered around the bed. She was looking at me with a friendly smile, and she seemed a little paler than she had when I came in.

"That's fine," I said.

She put the portfolio and the pictures away and lay with her hands clasped in front of her.

"Ready when you are," she said.

I examined her eyes, ears, and mouth; they were normal. As I felt her neck I noticed a strange texture under my fingers, and I bent over to look. Along the skin on the side of her neck were small, slightly raised, waxy-looking areas. I'd never seen anything like them before.

"Oh, those are amyloid," she said. "I've got more here." She hoisted up her nightgown and showed me a large cluster of similar spots under her right arm. "They are all over the place."

She was very matter-of-fact about it, pulling her nightgown back down. "Or do you need it up to listen to my lungs?"

"Actually, yes, thanks," I said. For some reason, seeing the spots had flustered me. She straightened and pulled up her nightgown. I held it up in back and listened to her lungs as she took deep breaths for me.

Her lungs sounded awful. They'd taken us to listen to

patients with congestive heart failure so we could hear what fluid in the lungs sounded like, but this was worse than anything I'd heard before. Her lungs sounded as if they were filled with fluid.

I quickly put the nightgown back down. "Could you lie down for me?" I asked.

She hesitated. "I can't lie flat very long—makes it hard for me to breathe. Can you be quick?"

"Sure," I said, wondering if I should be doing the exam at all. Maybe an extra physical wasn't such a great thing after all.

She pushed away the pillows and lay flat. I pulled up her nightgown enough to listen to her heart without exposing her breasts. I thought I might have heard an S4, the sound heard in heart failure, but I wasn't sure, and I didn't want to take the extra time to be sure.

I quickly moved down to her abdomen, pulling down the quilt. She was a heavy woman, but it was more than that; the puffiness that I'd seen in her face was apparent everywhere. As I probed her abdomen with the pads of my fingers, I found that her liver was huge, and hard. It must be full of amyloid, I thought. My hands shook a little.

"Almost done down there?" she asked. Her voice was a little weak.

I covered her abdomen with her nightgown, leaving the quilt down. "All done," I said. "You can sit up now."

She sat up, and I helped arrange the pillows behind her. She looked tired, and she was breathing more quickly than before.

"Are you okay?" I asked.

"I'll be fine," she said. "You finish up."

I did a brief exam of her legs and a quick neurological exam. I was enjoying it less and less. Her legs and feet were horribly swollen with extra fluid caused by her heart failure and probably her kidney failure as well. Her neuro exam showed that she was losing some of the sensation in her hands and feet. I remembered that amyloidosis could affect nerves, causing symptoms like these.

I covered her again with the quilt and looked at her. Meredith is not going to her daughter's wedding, I realized. Meredith isn't going to live that long.

I excused myself quickly, thanking her and saying that I was late to meet my instructor, which wasn't exactly true. I found it hard to look her in the eye or return her smile. I just wanted to get out of there.

I had been so entranced by the idea that my touch could be curative that it hadn't occurred to me that there might be someone for whom my touch would be uncomfortable and unhelpful. And somehow I had never thought about how I would feel, or what I would say, when I found something I didn't want to find—something serious and terrible in someone I liked.

I thought I was so equipped, so ready with my new knowledge, skills, and power. As I walked quickly down the hallway away from Meredith's room, my heart pounding, I realized that I wasn't ready at all. I felt ashamed that I hadn't known what to say or do, that all I'd done was run away.

The laying on of hands involved more than knowledge or cures or power, I realized. It involved things more fundamental and more difficult: acceptance, faith, and a kind of helping that I didn't really understand yet.

KNOWING
THE WORDS

I spoke some Spanish when I started medical school, but not much. I had taken it in high school and back then spoke it fairly well; I had some good teachers and a friend from Chile who made me speak it with her. But after that I used it very little; I took only one Spanish course my freshman year in college, and I lost touch with the friend from Chile. By the time I started medical school I had forgotten most of what I knew.

I began my third-year clerkships with Surgery. It was an ambitious start, as Surgery was a particularly difficult and important clerkship, but I wanted to jump right in with something demanding. I had been dreaming of these clerkships, of getting out of the classroom and into the hospitals full-time, and I was itching to be immersed and challenged.

The Surgery rotation was two months long, divided into one month on the general surgery wards, two weeks in the emergency room, one week of Anesthesia, and one week of elective in a surgical subspecialty. The month on the wards was considered the most crucial part. During that month you were assigned to a team of residents, and you did your best to become an integral part of that team. You were to go on rounds, help care for surgical patients, do as much in the operating room as you were allowed, and do any jobs the residents might give you. You were also expected to do a lot of reading from surgical textbooks. At any point during rounds or in the midst of an operation, a resident or more likely an attending surgeon might ask you to name all the layers of the abdominal wall, or all the possible positions of the appendix, or just about anything else—and you were expected to answer correctly.

There were three general surgery services at the Brigham and Women's Hospital. I was assigned to the Cushing Service, which was the ward service, the service for patients who didn't have a private doctor. They were mostly low-income patients from the inner-city neighborhoods around the Brigham, and many of them were Latino.

The Spanish vocabulary of the surgical residents was very limited. As far as I could tell, the only words they knew were *sí, no,* and *dolor,* the word for "pain." "*¿Dolor?*" they would ask as they pointed or poked at various parts of the patient. The patient would nod or shake his head. If he said anything else, they would generally ignore it. My limited Spanish skills became suddenly impressive. The fact that I could say "*¿Dónde le duele?*" ("Where does it hurt?") and at least sort of understand the answer made me practically fluent in the eyes of the surgical residents. I began to do some very basic translating for them. It made me feel useful and important, rare feelings for a third-year student. I didn't know many medical words, and I quickly got lost if the patient spoke fast or said a lot at once, but it didn't matter. The residents were a little nicer to me than they might otherwise have been, and I didn't feel so bad if I forgot one of the layers of the abdominal wall.

One night when I was on call we brought a patient to the intensive care unit to put in a central line, a special kind of IV. He was about seventy-five, from Guatemala, and the next day he was to have surgery on his blood vessels. His son had brought him to the hospital because he had been complaining of pains in his legs whenever he walked more than a short distance. The ward service resident ordered some tests, which showed that the major blood vessels leading into both of his legs were blocked, preventing adequate blood flow; this caused the pain. The resident explained to the son, who could speak English, that surgery could be done to correct the problem. It was major surgery, involving opening both of the legs and attaching synthetic grafts to the vessels to bypass the obstruction. The son explained to the old man, who spoke no English. The old man shrugged and said something I couldn't understand. The son told the resident that his father didn't care, but that he, the son, wanted him to have the surgery. He didn't like seeing his father in pain.

So the surgery was scheduled. A central line is an intravenous line that is placed into one of the large veins of the neck and threaded down until it is close to the heart. This allows for careful monitoring of the patient during and after the operation. It's a routine procedure, but because it's a little tricky, and dangerous if complications occur, it is done in the intensive care unit.

I was sent to get the patient. I found a wheelchair and went to the surgical ward. I told the nurse who I was and that I had come for Mr. Escobar. She nodded and pointed to one of the rooms. "He's in the first bed," she said.

Mr. Escobar was sitting on the chair next to his bed. The television was on, but he didn't seem to be watching it; his eyes were staring at nothing in particular. He looked as if he were remembering something, thinking about something from long ago.

He wore a faded plaid cotton shirt and worn blue cotton pants. His big, gnarled hands were folded in front of him, resting on his rounded belly. He had thick gray hair with a few streaks of black and strong, well-defined features. His wrinkled brown skin looked like the skin of someone who had spent most of his life outdoors. As he turned to look at me, his eyes were deep brown and calm.

"I am the medical student," I said in Spanish. "I have come to take you to the other floor." I didn't know how to say "intensive care unit"; I figured that since he had signed the consent for the central line, someone had explained to him what would happen and where he would need to go. He nodded and reached for the wooden cane that rested against the bedside table. "No," I said in Spanish. "I will take you in this." I pointed to the wheelchair. "You do not need to walk."

The old man frowned, then shrugged. I put the brakes on the wheelchair and helped him out of his chair and into it. As I began to back it out of the room, he reached for his cane again. Just in case, his eyes seemed to say to me. I smiled and handed it to him; he laid it across his lap.

I put his chart in the pocket on the back of the chair, and we started down the long hallway toward the elevators. I felt as though I should chat with him, but my limited vocabulary didn't allow much conversation. "For how many years have you lived here?" I asked in clumsy Spanish.

"*Cinco años,*" he said. Five years.

"What did you do there?"

"*Tenía finca,*" he said. ("I had a farm.") That explained his skin and his hands.

"Which do you prefer, the United States or Guatemala?"

The old man paused. He ran his fingers along his cane. "*Mi país,*" he said. ("My country.")

The elevator doors opened. I pushed the button to hold them open and backed him inside. The wheels caught in the space between the hallway floor and the bottom of the elevator. I had to pull hard to get them out, and as I did it jolted him forward. "I'm so sorry. I mean, *Lo siento,*" I said. I should have let him walk, I thought.

The old man looked at me and smiled. His eyes were kind. "*No te preocupes,*" he said. ("Don't worry.") He used the familiar *tú* form of the verb, the form that is used with friends or younger people. The more formal *usted* is usually used with doctors.

I released the hold button and pressed the button for the intensive care unit. When the doors opened again I wheeled him out very gently and carefully. This time it went smoothly. I wheeled him down to the intensive care unit and to the bed space the nurse pointed out. As I put the brakes on and helped him up, he nodded to me.

"*Gracias,*" he said.

"*De nada,*" I said. ("You're welcome.")

I found the surgical senior. I liked him more than other seniors I had met—most of them just made me nervous, made me feel as though I were always saying or doing the wrong thing. Bill didn't praise me or even routinely encourage me, but he made a point of including me in any patient examination or procedure that was interesting, and he ignored me just enough to take the pressure off me, but not so much that he didn't teach me anything.

Bill was reviewing the procedures for placing a central line with Ron, the junior resident. Ron was a thin, small, Asian man with big round glasses that overwhelmed his face. He was in his second year and was one of the most efficient residents in the program. He got more done than anyone on the surgical floors and still managed to spend a lot of time in the operating room. I think he did this by being constantly in motion and doing everything quickly—but never sloppily. He was a perfectionist. He was nice to the medical students, but catching him, literally stopping him to ask a question was difficult, and he ran out of patience quickly if the student didn't understand the answer immediately or had further questions.

Bill was sitting at the table in the small conference room, drinking coffee as he sketched the anatomy of the neck for Ron, who was standing next to him. Both wore wrinkled blue scrubs and white coats; both looked disheveled and tired. The surgical residents were on call every other night except for weekends, when they worked either both Thursday and Friday nights or Saturday and Sunday nights. The idea was to give the residents a weekend off every other week, but working sixty or so hours straight to do this seemed kind of crazy to me. The surgical residents probably thought it was crazy, too, but they put up with it and didn't complain. It was the initiation process; it was the culture.

"Mr. Escobar is here," I announced. They looked up at me. Bill smiled and nodded; Ron looked back down at Bill's drawing.

"So you like to approach this way?" he said, pointing. "Tim showed me a different way, and I've done it that way the other times."

Bill shrugged. "Do whatever feels comfortable," he said. "I'm just showing you the way I like to do it." He got up and walked toward Mr. Escobar's bedside. Ron picked up the drawing, put it in his pocket, and walked after him. I followed, wondering if I should keep a certain number of paces behind.

Mr. Escobar was in the bed. He had changed into a hospital gown, one of the standard blue-and-white ones that don't cover well. I felt embarrassed for him somehow and moved to the bed to pull up the covers. He took them from me and nodded. His eyes were questioning.

"He does understand what you guys are going to do, doesn't he?" I asked Bill.

Bill shrugged. "The consent's signed," he said.

I picked up the chart and flipped through it until I found the consent form, the standard form for a surgical procedure with blanks for filling in the exact procedure to be done and for listing any special risks.

"This is in English," I said.

"His son translated," said Ron.

I had watched the son translate in that first conversation about the surgery. He had his own ideas about what should happen to his father and may have edited the consent so that his father wouldn't say no. He had certainly edited when they talked about the surgery. My Spanish wasn't good enough to understand everything he was saying, but it was good enough to know that he was leaving out some things that the surgeons had said. I didn't say anything at the time; I felt it wasn't my place. Maybe the son had been more honest with the consent. Somehow, though, I doubted it.

"Do you understand what they are going to do?" I asked the old man in Spanish.

"*Mi hijo dijo algo, pero no me recuerdo. Algo pequeño que hay que hacer antes de la cirugía, creo que dijo,*" said the man. ("I don't remember exactly what my son said, but I think it was something about a small thing that they have to do before the surgery.")

I suppose that in comparison with the upcoming surgery, the placement of a central line was small, but I don't know that I would have described it that way. He would have to lie very still with his head to one side while a needle was put into a vein in his neck. Then he would have to keep lying still while they threaded the catheter down through the vein and sewed some sutures into his skin to keep it in place. They would use local anesthetic, but it was going to be uncomfortable and probably frightening.

The old man must have sensed something from my expression. "*¿Porqué? ¿Qué van a hacer?*" he said. ("Why? What are they going to do?")

I wanted to explain, to tell him everything, but I didn't know the words. How could I say it? They are going to put a big IV into your neck—but I didn't know the words for "IV" or "neck." I couldn't say "needle," I couldn't say "sutures," I couldn't say "anesthetic." I hadn't learned those words in high school—they hadn't come up in the Spanish literature we'd read.

"Could we call an interpreter?" I asked.

"Why?" asked Ron. "The consent's signed, isn't it?"

"Yes," I said, "but I don't think he knows what's happening."

"Look, it's late, and we need to get on with this," said Ron. "I'm sure his son explained everything. If we run into problems, we'll call the interpreter."

I looked at Bill; he shrugged. A good senior never interfered unless it was absolutely necessary. He let the junior run things whenever possible so that he or she would learn to take charge. Clearly he didn't consider this important enough to overrule Ron.

The old man was looking at me. I had not answered his question.

"They are going to do something that they have to do before the surgery, as your son said," I said in Spanish. "But it isn't really small. It's important, but it isn't small. I don't know the words to explain it, I'm sorry." I felt horrible. I tried to imagine what it would be like to be lying there, hearing so many words and knowing they were about me and what was going to happen to me but not being able to understand them.

The nurse lowered the head of the bed. She took his head gently and turned it toward her, exposing the right side of his neck to Ron, who had put on a mask, a surgical gown, and sterile gloves. He cleaned the skin carefully with Betadine and laid sterile blue cloths across the man's face and shoulder so that the neck, the "sterile field," was defined. The old man was still. Ron picked up the syringe with local anesthetic and inserted the needle underneath the skin in the middle of the field.

The old man reached up with his big hand and grabbed Ron's arm, pushing it away from his neck. "No," he said.

"Shit," Ron said under his breath. "Now we have to start all over again." Once the field or his gown was touched by something nonsterile, such as Mr. Escobar's hand, it was contaminated and the risk of infection was higher. He took off the gloves and gown and put on new ones. The nurse, Bill, and I stood quietly.

Ron reached for the Betadine and started to clean the neck again. Mr. Escobar sat up. He took the nurse by surprise, and she was unable to stop him. "No," he said.

"Mr. Escobar, we have to do this," said Ron, loudly and sternly.

Mr. Escobar's brown eyes were almost black with anger, and his hands were clenched in whitened fists. "No," he said. "*Déjame en paz.*"

Ron looked at me. "What'd he say?"

"He wants you to leave him alone," I said.

"This is just great," said Ron. He turned to Bill. "Now what are we going to do? Sedate him? Tie him down?"

I looked at my watch. "It's only eight-thirty," I said. "I'm sure we can get an interpreter now. Maybe if he understood what was going on, he'd be cooperative."

"Why don't you explain it to him?" asked Ron. "You speak Spanish."

So much for being impressive, I thought. "Not well enough," I said.

Ron looked at Bill. "I don't think we have a lot of choice," said Bill. "We would need general anesthesia to keep this guy still, and I don't want to tie him down."

"I'll page the interpreter," said the nurse. She looked at me gratefully.

About ten minutes later the interpreter arrived. She was a young woman, nicely dressed, with long black hair tied back in a scarf. "I'm Marta Ramirez," she said. "What do you need?"

Bill and Ron were leaning against the counter a few feet away, talking. "I'm the medical student," I said. "We need to put a central line into Mr. Escobar here. I tried to explain, but my Spanish wasn't good enough." She looked at me with something like disdain and walked over to Mr. Escobar's bedside. She introduced herself to him, and the two of them began to talk; I recognized her accent as Puerto Rican. Mr. Escobar was very animated, gesturing angrily. Marta's voice was calm, soothing, direct. I stood as close behind her as I could without being rude. I wanted to hear what she was saying. I couldn't understand everything, but I could make out enough to figure out some of the words I hadn't known; *suero* was IV, *aguja* was needle, *anestesia* was anesthetic.

Marta turned to me and to the surgeons, who had come over to watch. "He'll go ahead with it," she said. "He's not happy about it, but he'll do it."

Ron went over to the bedside table, where the nurse had laid out sterile gloves, another gown, and fresh sterile cloths. He put on a mask, looking uncertainly at Bill, who was putting on gloves, too, so he could hand Ron things he needed during the procedure. Marta went over to the side of the bed where the nurse was standing and pulled up a chair. As Ron cleaned and draped she explained in Spanish everything he was doing. I listened intently, memorizing every word I could.

"I'm going to put in the anesthetic now," said Ron. "He better not move."

Marta looked up at Ron. She seemed annoyed. "*Se va a poner la aguja con el anestésico,*" she said to Mr. Escobar. "*No se mueva.*"

Ron carefully placed the needle under the skin. He hesitated a moment, but Mr. Escobar didn't move. He pushed in the local anesthetic. "It's going to burn a little," he said.

"*Va a arder un poco,*" Marta said to Mr. Escobar.

Ron went on with the procedure. With each step he announced what he was about to do and what Mr. Escobar might feel, and Marta translated. I was surprised; I had watched Ron do other procedures, including central lines, and usually he didn't say anything to the patient, let alone give explanations or warnings. Usually he just did it.

Bill didn't say much. He stood by, handing Ron the guide wire, catheter, suture, and other things he needed. Every once in a while he'd say "Good" or "That's right." Ron was deft at procedures like this one and didn't need much guidance. Bill's eyes were fixed on Ron's hands and the part of Mr. Escobar's neck where Ron was working. He seemed to ignore Marta and the ongoing translations. Soon Ron was finished. The blue cloths were removed, Ron took off his gown, and Marta left. Mr. Escobar lay very still on the hospital bed, his eyes gazing out the window. I wanted to apologize, I wanted to explain about the procedure and the surgery and about the way surgeons act sometimes. I wanted to say so much, but I didn't know the words.

The next day after evening rounds, when I could finally leave the hospital, I went over to the bookstore and bought a textbook of medical Spanish. For the rest of my surgical clerkship, I studied vocabulary lists every night along with the different approaches to gallbladder removal or the causes of small bowel obstruction.

Suddenly it seemed to me that it wasn't good enough to know a lot of information or be deft at procedures. Suddenly it seemed to me that to really take care of people, you had to be able to communicate with them, to help them understand what was happening to them and allow them to become involved. It didn't seem fair to deprive people of this communication just because they didn't speak English. I couldn't learn every language and communicate with everyone, but I could learn Spanish.

Mr. Escobar's surgery went well, and it wasn't long before he was pacing the halls with his cane. He walked with a sort of wonderment; that his pain was gone must have seemed a miracle to him. I checked on him every day and practiced new words. He seemed to understand what I was doing and was pleasantly patient with my hesitations and mistakes.

The day he left the hospital, he refused to ride in a wheelchair to the lobby; he insisted on walking by himself. His son and I walked close by, carrying his bags. As we reached the lobby doors I handed what I was carrying to his son and turned to Mr. Escobar.

"*Buena suerte,*" I said. ("Good luck.")

He smiled gently and took my hand. "*Y a ti también,*" he said. ("And to you, too.")

INSIDES

She lay on the stretcher in the emergency room and described her symptoms, which were classic. It was as if she had memorized them from a textbook. First she had a stomachache, although it wasn't a particularly bad one, and then she lost her appetite. A few hours later the stomachache grew much worse.

"Where in your stomach did it hurt?" asked Bill.

She grimaced as she adjusted herself on the stretcher. "It started here," she said, pointing to somewhere around her belly button. "But now it hurts more here." She pointed to the lower part of her abdomen, on the right.

Bill looked over at me, to be sure I was paying attention.

She was slender, with chin-length blond hair and bangs, fair skin, and a nose that was sort of large but somehow looked good on her; she was pretty. She looked to be in her early twenties, about my age. I felt a little awkward, the way I always did when the patient was my age. It was easier when they were younger or older. When they were my age I felt like they saw through me, like they knew I was a student and unsure of myself.

"Any nausea or vomiting?" asked Bill. "Any change in your stools? Pain when you urinate? Fever? Vaginal discharge?"

She frowned, as if she were having trouble remembering all the questions. "Some nausea, I guess. And I think the nurse said I had a little fever. Nothing else."

Bill looked over at the nursing sheet where the vital signs were written. I looked over his shoulder. Her temperature was 100.9.

"Hmm," said Bill. He washed his hands at the small sink in the examining room, dried them on a paper towel, and went over to the stretcher.

"I'm going to examine you, okay?"

"Okay," she said, but she looked nervous. She looked up at the man who was with her. He was tall and thin and wore a Boston University T-shirt and jeans; he seemed to be her boyfriend. He put his hand on her shoulder and nodded. It's okay, he seemed to say.

Bill pulled a sheet out of the cabinet and laid it over her legs up to her pelvis, then pulled up the hospital gown so he could see her abdomen. It was a nice gesture; without the sheet she would have been lying there in just her underpants. I'm not sure she appreciated it, but I did. It's not always easy for a tired and harried surgical senior to be thoughtful.

Bill rubbed his hands together to warm them a little and then reached over with his right hand. She watched him closely. Gently, expertly, he pressed on her abdomen with his fingers and the upper part of his palm. He watched her face as he pressed.

"Some voluntary guarding," he said without turning to look at me. That meant that she was tensing her abdominal muscles to prevent him from pushing in too deep, something that people with abdominal pain often do.

She looked over toward me, to see whom he was talking to. I think it was the first time she had realized I was in the room. I nodded hello and she nodded back. She looked at me questioningly, but not very intently. It was as if she wanted to know who I was, but she was too uncomfortable to care very much. I wondered if I should introduce myself; I had been hoping that Bill would say, as he usually did, "This is the medical student working with me"—but he didn't.

She looked back at Bill. The opportunity was lost; I didn't introduce myself.

Bill was slowly moving his hand across the different parts of her abdomen, trying to find exactly where it was most tender. It seemed to bother her somewhat everywhere; she kept wincing. But when he pressed on the right side of her lower abdomen, she jumped.

"Ow! There, that's where it hurts the most."

Bill turned toward me. "Right lower quadrant," he said. He turned back to her and pressed there again.

"Ow! Please stop, that really hurts."

The boyfriend took a step closer, as if to put himself between her and Bill. Bill took a step back.

"Okay, okay," he said. "I just had to be sure."

He motioned me toward the door. "We'll be right back," he said.

I followed him out into the late evening bustle of the emergency room. He found two chairs in a noisy corner, and we sat down. The emergency room doctor who had seen the woman first had done a full physical exam, including a pelvic exam, and had drawn blood for tests. We looked at what she had written about the woman's exam and the results of the tests. We discussed the "differential diagnosis," all the possible conditions the woman might have that would cause her symptoms. He quizzed me, made me run through them all and say why I thought each was more or less likely.

"So, what do you think she's got?" he said when I had run through what he felt was an adequately exhaustive list of possibilities.

"Appendicitis."

He smiled. "So do I. So what do we do?"

"Take her to the operating room."

"But what if we're wrong? What if she's just got the flu?" he said with his eyebrows up, prompting me.

"Better to operate and be wrong than to miss an appendicitis that ends up perforated," I said. This was what we had been taught in our teaching sessions.

"Right. And sometimes when it's not appendicitis it's something else that needs to be operated on anyway, so it's good that we're in there."

He pulled himself out of the chair and went to look for a surgical consent form. Despite the long years of medical school and surgical residency, and a few extra pounds, he still had a football player's build. One of the other residents had told me that he was quite a star in college. He moved more slowly and comfortably than the other surgical residents, unless of course there was an emergency.

I went back into the room with him and listened as he explained to the woman and her boyfriend why he thought it was appendicitis and why he thought it was important that we take her to the operating room that night. The woman bit her lip and stared into Bill's eyes as he spoke. Her shoulders tensed as he discussed the possible risks of the operation, such as bleeding or infection. Her boyfriend reached for her hand and held it.

"Any questions?" asked Bill. The woman shook her head.

"Will you be doing the operation?" asked the boyfriend.

"Yes," said Bill, "with one of the other surgeons, Dr. Alber, assisting me."

He didn't mention me. In a way I was glad, because he would have had to say that I was a student, and she probably didn't want a student, especially one her age, taking part in her operation; still, I was going to be there in the operating room, and it felt a little strange not to be mentioned.

"You need to sign this," said Bill, holding out the surgical consent form. The woman took it and started to read it. "Let me get you a pen."

"Here," I said, pulling a pen out of my pocket. Her boyfriend let go of her hand and took a step back as I brought it over to her. She took it and thanked me. We looked at each other for a moment; I smiled nervously, and she returned the smile, politely. She signed the form; Alice Hampton, she wrote in neat script. She handed the form to Bill and gave me the pen.

Bill paged Victor Alber, the surgical intern, and told him where to meet us. He spoke with Alice's nurse and made a few phone calls to make all the arrangements necessary for the operation. I couldn't find a chair, so I sat on the edge of the counter, trying not to stare at Alice Hampton and her boyfriend. He was rubbing her shoulders and talking to her. She lay there with her hands on her abdomen, looking scared. She glanced up while I was staring at her, and our eyes met. Embarrassed, I got up off the counter and walked around the emergency room until Bill was ready to leave.

Victor was waiting for us in the lounge outside the operating room suite. He was short and dark, with a five o'clock shadow that seemed always to be there, even when he had clearly just shaved. He always looked tired, too, but that was understandable; the first-year residents, who are called interns, work incredibly long hours. He was nice, but he was usually too busy to pay much attention to me.

He was sitting on one of the armchairs, his feet up on a nearby table. "Hey," he said to Bill, and nodded hello to me. "An appy, huh?"

"Sure looks like one," said Bill, sitting down. He leaned back, his hands behind his head. "Done any since you started internship?"

"One," said Victor. "But I did a few as a student."

Bill reviewed the procedure and technique with him. I sat on a chair near Bill's and looked around the room. I looked longingly at the vending machines. I hadn't eaten dinner, and I was really hungry.

"You listening?" said Bill. I realized he was talking to me.

"Yes," I said, sitting up straight.

He explained and drew on the back of a napkin exactly how to remove an appendix. Victor seemed to know what to do. We got up and went into the suite of operating rooms, put on our shoe covers, masks, and hats, and scrubbed our hands and forearms in the big sinks. I watched them closely and imitated the way they scrubbed and the way they backed themselves into the operating room with their hands up in the air to keep them clean. When the circulating nurse was finished with Bill and Victor, she helped me put on sterile gloves and a sterile gown to cover my scrubs. It was only the second time I had been in the operating room, so it was all still very unfamiliar. I felt like an outsider in some sort of closed society. Everybody seemed to know exactly what to do but me.

The room was big and bright and bare, except for the operating table, two smaller tables covered with instruments, and various stools, some for sitting and some for standing. The walls were yellow, and metal supply cabinets with glass doors lined two of them. It was cold; I shivered under the paper gown, wishing for something warmer.

Alice lay on the operating table in the middle of the room, covered from the neck down by a sheet. She had been brought in while we were scrubbing. The anesthesiologist had already put her to sleep and put a breathing tube down her windpipe so that he could control her breathing and keep her asleep. Leads were running from her chest to a monitor that recorded her heart and respiratory rates; it beeped and had wavy lines running across its screen. Her hair was gathered under a paper cap to keep it out of the way. Her skin looked pale and yellow under the big, adjustable bright lights that hung over the table. The breathing tube was secured to her face with adhesive tape so that it wouldn't come out. Her eyes were closed, and she was very still.

Victor pulled down the sheet that covered her and washed her abdomen with Betadine, moving in small to larger circles, several times. Her abdomen was flat, with nice muscular lines; it looked as though she did lots of sit-ups. She is probably proud of it, I thought; she probably always wears bikinis to the beach. I looked at Victor and Bill, trying to catch some expression on their faces under the masks, some reaction to the fact that there was a very pretty naked woman lying on the table in front of them. I didn't see anything. In the operating room things are different, I was finding out, but it was a hard transition for me to make. I still felt like the same person I had been when I was out there scrubbing my hands in the sink or in the emergency room, listening to Alice and watching her with her boyfriend. Bill and Victor, somehow, were different people.

Victor laid the sterile cloths across her pelvis and upper abdomen, to define the area to be operated on and create the sterile field. When they were placed we took our positions: Bill and I were on one side, Victor was on the other. The scrub nurse stood on a stool by the draped table covered with surgical instruments; she was gloved and gowned as we were, and her job was to hand the surgeons the instrument or suture they needed at any given time.

Under Bill's direction, Victor took a scalpel from the scrub nurse and made an incision in the right lower quadrant of Alice's abdomen. He cut through the skin, down to the muscle, and then through that into the abdominal cavity. He was neat and careful; it was a straight incision, and there was very little bleeding. Nevertheless, I shuddered and resisted an urge to put my hand over that part of my abdomen.

Bill must have noticed my shudder. "Don't worry," he said. "The incision is mostly below the bikini line." That wasn't what I was shuddering about, I thought.

All of Alice's body was covered except for the part of her abdomen outlined by the cloths. Her legs were covered, her chest was covered, her head was behind a low curtain so that the anesthesiologist could do his work without getting in the way of the surgeons. It's like she's just an abdomen now, I thought.

Bill put a retractor into the incision and handed it to me. I pulled back on the long handle and stretched open the incision, making it easier for Victor to see what he was doing. Under Bill's direction, Victor reached in with his fingers and began to pull out the underlying intestine, looking for the appendix.

"There's the cecum," said Bill, pointing to a pouchlike structure at the junction between the small and large intestine.

"And here's the appendix," said Victor, holding a small bit of intestine that looked like a worm hanging off the cecum. "Doesn't really look all that inflamed."

"Doesn't look quite normal either, though. Let's take it off."

I watched as Victor cut and sutured. In a few minutes the appendix was off.

"While we're here, since that didn't look all that awful, let's run the bowel," said Bill, meaning he wanted to look at the rest of the intestine to be sure they weren't missing something.

I pulled harder on the retractor to open the incision a little more, and Victor went in with his fingers and started pulling out intestine. I watched with amazement as more and more of it lay outside her abdomen. Bill ran over it with his thumb and index finger, looking for abnormalities. It all seemed fine.

Finally Bill and Victor finished. They stopped and looked down at the intestine lying on the skin. It was disturbing to me. Intestine was supposed to be inside, not outside. Skin and muscle were there for a reason; they contained and covered things that weren't meant to be seen. I tried to concentrate only on the intestine. We are looking for an abnormality, I told myself. Do not think about Alice's face or the way her boyfriend touched her in the emergency room. Do not even think about how the rest of her body is lying here. Just think about this incision and whether or not this intestine looks normal.

"Okay, Claire," said Bill. "Put it back in."

"What?" I asked, dumbfounded.

"You heard what I said. Put it back in."

Victor looked at me and smiled behind his mask.

"How?" I asked.

"Just put it in," said Bill. "Nothing complicated about it." He took the retractor from me.

I reached over with my gloved hands and touched her

intestine. It was warm and squishy. Carefully I picked up part of one end of the long loop and slowly put it back in the incision, pushing it in as deep into her abdominal cavity as I could. Then I picked up the next section of the loop and did the same, just as carefully.

"We'll be here all night, Claire," said Bill. "Just put it in."

Nervously, my hands shaking, I began pushing it in a few centimeters at a time, as fast as I could. I thought they would tell me I was doing it too quickly, but instead they acted impatient. I was frightened that I was doing it wrong, that it was going to end up in the wrong place or twisted or folded in on itself, that she was going to have an obstruction in her intestine or some other problem because of me. I kept thinking Bill or Victor would stop me, tell me to do something differently, but they watched without comment.

While doing dissection in Anatomy, I had touched intestine, but it was cold, not this pliable, and besides, the person was dead; I couldn't do any damage, and it didn't feel like such an invasion of privacy. This woman was alive, and I felt very awkward to be touching her this way. Even after months of Anatomy and Physiology I found it difficult to be purely clinical. They were still "insides," like we called them when we were children, and it made me very uncomfortable to touch them.

Finally I finished.

"Fine," said Bill. "Thank you. Victor, please close."

As Victor carefully sewed the various layers back together and then stapled the skin, I watched him and slowly calmed down enough to stop shaking.

The next day on afternoon rounds we went by to see Alice. She was sitting up in bed; her boyfriend was sitting by her feet, and they were smiling and talking animatedly when we came in. Her blond hair was pulled back in a short ponytail, and she looked pale but otherwise well. I was relieved. I figured that if I had done something bad when I put her intestine back in, she would have had symptoms by then.

"How do you feel?" asked Bill.

"Okay, I guess," she said. I stood behind Victor, out of view.

"We got the report back from the pathologist who looked at your appendix after we took it out," said Bill. "It was very inflamed. Definitely appendicitis."

So we didn't need to do all that, I thought. They didn't need to pull out all that intestine and make me put it back in. Even though I knew we were being safe and thorough by doing so, I felt all the more awkward.

Victor leaned over to tie his shoelace, and suddenly Alice looked right at me; I squirmed. I touched your insides, I wanted to blurt out, I hope you don't mind.

I didn't say anything, and she looked away.

Bill started talking about pain medicine and when she could go home. Victor stood up again, and I took my place behind him.

SOMETHING
TO DO

*I*t was late, or at least it felt late. I was taking overnight call with the residents as part of my gynecology
clerkship at Massachusetts General Hospital. I'd finished
my clerkships in surgery, pediatrics, and radiology, so I felt
much more comfortable with the routines of the hospital.
The residents had kept me busy that night with the tradi-
tional on-call jobs of the third-year student: putting in IVs,
drawing blood, hunting down lab results, doing admission
physicals, and writing up admission notes. We took that
work very seriously as students. It was our chance to shine
and impress people, something it was very important to do
as a third-year student. We needed to get good grades and
written evaluations in order to be accepted into competitive
residency programs.

But it was frustrating; we wanted more. After two years
of lectures and studying and tests, we were ready to do something important, to begin to be doctors instead of just doing
what the residents called "scut work." Every once in a while
we would have an opportunity: perhaps there would be an

emergency, and the IV that we put in quickly while everyone else was busy was the one that lifesaving medications were given through; perhaps the resident would let us do a procedure such as putting a chest tube into someone whose lung had collapsed or sticking a needle into someone's abdomen to remove extra fluid, called ascites. We were always watching for these opportunities to play a crucial role.

It felt late, but it was only around eleven. My feet were tired, and the day had been long and depressing. I'd spent the morning on seemingly endless rounds and the afternoon in the operating room, holding retractors for hours during a hysterectomy while the gynecologist doing the surgery snapped at me intermittently for not holding them the way he wanted me to. Both of the admissions I had done in the evening were young women with ovarian cancer, one of whom bore a disturbing resemblance to a friend of mine.

The senior resident, a generally pleasant and gentle woman in her early thirties, was hassled and exhausted, not in the mood to spend any extra time with a medical student. She sat across from me at the desk at the nurses' station, making notes on index cards about the patients who had been admitted and what would need to be done for them the following day. The intern was doing the rest of the admissions and the last work of the day—checking once more on the patients and their lab results, writing any last progress notes and orders. She was a surgical intern doing a rotation on the gynecology service, a thin, frenetic woman in her late twenties who was too busy to talk to me. Our only contact throughout the evening had been the times she'd paged me to ask me to draw yet another person's blood.

I wanted to go home, or at least curl up in the cramped, dingy call room and go to sleep. But I had the finishing touches to do on my second admission note. I had to be sure that my assessment section was well written and com-

plete, that I hadn't left out any diagnostic possibility or com-
plicating factor, and I had to be sure that the plan, the last
part of the note, contained everything that should or might
be done with the patient. The admission notes were read by
the residents and the attendings and played a role in our
grade, so we did our best to make them perfect. Besides, it
was too early to go to sleep. The later you stayed up, the
better, we thought. If you went to sleep too early, the residents might think you were uninterested or lazy.

The senior's beeper went off. She sighed, fumbled for it
under the sweater she wore over her green scrubs, hit the
button, and called the operator. It was the emergency room.
After pulling out a blank index card, she dialed the number.
"Gynecology, answering a page," she said.

I was excited. This could mean something interesting, this
could mean something to do. It was especially good when
emergencies happened at night, because fewer residents were
around, which meant the medical students might actually be
needed. Maybe we would have to take the patient to the
operating room; maybe I would be able to do some small
part of the operation, instead of just holding retractors.

"Okay," the senior resident was saying as she took notes
on the index card. "How old did you say she is? . . . Okay.
And how much bleeding? . . . I see. You have an IV in, right?
. . . Thanks. . . . Fine. I'll be down in a few minutes. Could
you do me a favor? Page my intern and tell her to meet me
there. Thanks." She hung up the phone, put the index card
in the shirt pocket of her scrubs along with all the others,
picked up her stethoscope, and headed toward the elevator.
I got up and walked after her. "Can I come?" I asked.

"Oh, yes, of course," said the senior, smiling apologeti-
cally. She had clearly forgotten about me. There was an awkward silence as we got into the elevator. "What does the
patient have?" I asked finally.

"It's a twenty-three-year-old woman who is having a miscarriage—seems like she's somewhere around sixteen weeks, judging from when her last period was. From the sound of it I don't think there is anything we can do to stop the miscarriage—she has been bleeding heavily for a few hours, probably passed the fetus. She needs a D and C."

Dilation and curettage—that's when the cervix is dilated and the uterus is scraped clean. "Why does she need that, if she has already passed the fetus?" I asked. It seemed to me that having a miscarriage was bad enough without going through having your uterus scraped clean.

The elevator doors opened, letting us out on the first floor. I followed the senior through the white hallway lined with stretchers and equipment that led to the emergency room. "We need to be sure that all the fetal material, including the placenta, has passed," she said. "Otherwise, there is a risk of infection. Also, the D and C can make the bleeding slow down, and from what they told me on the phone, she's lost a lot of blood."

We turned left out of the back corridors into the nighttime bustle of the emergency room. We had come the back way into its entrance area, with its big main desk to our right and in front of us the swinging doors that opened out to the street and the ambulance bays. Off to the left was the "triage" area, where patients were seen when they first arrived. If they came in by ambulance clearly very sick or injured, they went through triage very quickly or not at all. Otherwise they waited, some of them a long time. That night the triage area was full. There was a lot of noise: patients talking, some drunk ones yelling, the people at the desk answering the always ringing phones and making announcements over the loudspeaker, doctors and nurses discussing patients and making phone calls.

I followed the senior as she turned right into the doctors'

lounge, where the intern was sitting drinking coffee out of a Styrofoam cup. The room was otherwise empty except for the day's clutter. The round table in the middle was covered with sections of the day's newspapers, and there was an open pizza box with two dried-out pieces left. Textbooks, journals, and jackets were scattered on the chairs.

The intern looked tired, but she always looked that way. She was tall, with very short brown hair and brown eyes that could be either piercing or glazed over, depending on the amount of sleep she'd had. She wore the same green scrubs as the senior, but hers hung loosely over her skinny arms and legs. She wore a white coat over her scrubs; its pockets were filled with bits of paper, pocket-size surgical reference manuals, and random small surgical instruments. I think she wanted everyone to know she was a surgical intern doing a rotation on the gynecology service, not a gynecology intern. She was very proud of being one of only two women admitted to the surgical program. Although it was only a few months into her internship, she had already adopted the brusque, no-nonsense manner that many of the surgeons had. Since she's a surgeon, I thought, she probably won't want to do a D & C; it's not exactly a surgical procedure. Maybe I'll get to do it.

She jumped up from her chair when she saw us. "I got the message you wanted me down here. They didn't tell me much—some woman miscarrying? What does she need, a D and C?"

"Yep," said the senior. "Ever done one?"

"No," said the intern. "But I'd like to." My heart sank.

"Great," said the senior. "I'll lead you through it."

They both looked at me. "You can help," said the senior.

We wound our way past the confusion into the back hallway of the emergency room, a long corridor lined with examination rooms, most of them with several stretchers apiece. One of the emergency room residents saw us and pointed to a room toward the end. "In there," he said. "Bed space four. The GYN room is free, too. Let me know what you need."

The room he had pointed to had four stretchers, two on each side, separated by curtains. It was windowless and a little dark. The woman was on the stretcher in the far corner. She was probably of average height, but on the stretcher she looked small. She wore a faded blue hospital gown and lay very still on her back, staring at the plastic IV tubing that ran from the bag of clear fluid above her to her left hand, where adhesive tape held the catheter firmly into her vein. She had shoulder-length light brown hair that fell in tangled curls against the hospital pillow. Her skin looked as white as the sheet that covered her. Her features were soft, and as she turned to look at us I was startled by her eyes. They were big, blue, very wide, and scared.

The senior approached and put her hand on the woman's shoulder. I liked the senior more for it; I was disturbed by the woman's eyes. I think the intern was, too, because she stood back rather than jumping in to talk or examine, which would have been more her style. The two of us listened as the senior took the history.

Yes, she had known she was pregnant. It was the first time she had been pregnant, and she hadn't known how she felt about it at first since she and her boyfriend hadn't planned it; but the more she thought about it, the more she wanted the baby, so she didn't get an abortion, and she'd had one visit with an obstetrician. Everything was fine then, and from what the obstetrician had said, she was four months along now. That morning she had started to have some cramping, but she didn't think too much of it until the afternoon, when it got worse and she'd noticed some blood in her underwear. It wasn't much, and she'd heard that sometimes you can get some bleeding when you're pregnant, so she'd tried not to worry. Then all of a sudden the cramps got horrible and the bleeding got very heavy, and, well, not just blood was coming out.

The woman's voice broke, and she stopped talking. She closed her eyes and covered them with her hand, the one that didn't have an IV in it.

"What was coming out?" the senior asked softly. The intern and I stood very still.

"I don't know, I could have been wrong, there was so much blood in the toilet, but I thought I saw part of something . . . I didn't look closely. I—I couldn't." She began to cry silently, her shoulders shaking.

"It's okay," said the senior. "We understand." She rubbed her shoulder gently and told her what she had told me about the D & C and why it was important to do it. She asked a few more questions about medical history and allergies and medications. The woman mumbled her answers: No, nothing, no problems.

"Fine," said the senior. "Okay. We're going to go get things ready—it will just be a few minutes." She looked at the intern. "You come with me—I'll show you where everything is. Claire, you stay here, and ask any other questions you'd like." The two of them left. I stood motionless in my place; the woman lay with her eyes closed.

Other questions? About what? Was I supposed to ask her more about the bleeding, like exactly how much? Was I supposed to ask about the thing in the toilet, ask her to describe it in more detail? I didn't think she wanted to talk about it, and I didn't really want to hear about it, either. I took a step closer to the stretcher.

"How are you feeling?" I asked. That was stupid, I thought. Of course she feels horrible, and now I am going to make her notice it even more.

She opened her eyes and looked at me; she tried to smile just a little. "I've felt better. Are you the medical student?"

I smiled nervously. "Is it that obvious?"

"It's okay," she said. "My brother is a medical student."

"Does your family live around here?" I asked.

"No," she said. She closed her eyes and winced in pain.

"I'm sorry," I said. "We don't have to talk—I can leave you alone." I took a step away.

"No, it's okay, don't go," she said, opening her eyes again. "Talking gets my mind off it a little. My family lives in Detroit. I'm going to school here."

"What are you studying?"

"Psychology. I'm going for my master's." She winced again. I didn't know if I should say something about her wincing or not. Since I didn't know what to say, I decided not to.

"Does your boyfriend know this is happening?"

"No," she said. She paused. "We broke up, actually. He wasn't interested in being a father—he wanted me to get an abortion." She looked away; we were both silent.

The senior came back into the room with a wheelchair. "We're ready," she said. The woman sat up, and we helped her off the stretcher into the wheelchair. I carried the IV bag, holding it up as we wheeled her down the hall to the gynecology procedure room.

The room was tiny, only about ten feet square. It held an examining table with stirrups and a few cabinets stocked with various instruments and supplies. There wasn't room for much else, let alone all of us. I wondered if they might reconsider having me help. The intern stood in the corner, drawing medications out of little bottles into syringes. I stood aside while the senior helped the woman onto the table and gave her a sheet to cover herself. I handed the senior the IV bag, which she hung on the pole in the corner behind the table. She motioned to me to take the wheelchair out into the hall to make more room. I leaned up against the wall, trying to be as small as possible.

The senior explained the various instruments to the intern and showed her how to lay them out in the order in which she would need them. I looked at the woman; her eyes were widening again. I wished there were a way of teaching telepathically, so that patients wouldn't know that the doctor who was about to do something to them had never done it before.

"Your job, Claire," said the senior, "is to be the anesthesiologist." She handed me three syringes. "Versed, Fentanyl, saline flush. Okay?" I nodded. This was good; they needed me to do something.

They put the woman's feet into the stirrups. "Okay, Claire, give the Versed." I looked for a "port," a tiny branch off the IV tubing with a rubber end used for injecting medicines into the tubing. I found one close to where the IV entered her hand. I gave the Versed the way I had been taught: clamp the tubing above the port, swab the port with an alcohol wipe, insert the needle of the syringe through the port, carefully and slowly push the contents of the syringe into the tubing, repeat with some of the saline so that the medicine was pushed into the bloodstream and didn't stay in the tubing, then undo the clamp. I made sure I did it perfectly, although neither of them was watching. The Versed was meant to relax the woman, and she did seem to breathe more slowly and regularly. She lay very still, staring at the ceiling.

"Okay, now the Fentanyl," said the senior. This was the narcotic. The dose the senior handed me wouldn't put her to sleep, but it was enough to dull any pain significantly. I injected it the same way, again as perfectly as I could. I put the empty syringes into the needle box on the wall behind me.

They waited a few minutes, quietly, for the anesthetics to take effect. Then they began to work, the senior guiding the intern. They injected some local anesthetic into the cervix and inserted the dilators. "Does this hurt?" asked the senior. The woman shook her head, but she was biting her lip.

I stood there against the wall. What was I supposed to do now? The anesthetics were given; she might need more later, but not for a while. They had everything they needed laid neatly out for them within reach. There was no room at the foot of the table for me to get behind them, so I couldn't even watch. I wished the intern hadn't wanted to do the procedure. I imagined myself there instead of her, masterfully handling the instruments as the senior commented, "Good technique, Claire."

The senior began to explain to the intern how to scrape out the lining of the uterus. The woman stiffened and held on tightly to the sides of the table. I realized how awful the instructions sounded. She looked so pale, so frightened. I stood watching her for a few moments. Suddenly I realized what I could do.

I reached over and put my hand on hers. "You can squeeze my hand if you want," I said.

She looked at me. She didn't say anything, but she nodded ever so slightly and let go of the side of the table. I took her hand in mine; she squeezed it, hard.

I reached over with my other hand and pulled the trash can with its metal lid close enough for me to sit on it, so that I would be closer to eye level with her. As the intern worked, asking questions as she went along, I asked the woman about her classes. I felt stupid as soon as I asked. Surely she wouldn't want to talk, let alone about school. But the woman's eyes relaxed a little, and she answered readily. In short sentences interrupted by wincing, she listed her classes for me and said she was having trouble with her statistics course. Each time she winced she squeezed my hand a little harder.

It didn't seem very long before the senior was saying, "Okay, we're all done," taking the woman's feet out of the stirrups, and giving her instructions about what medicine to take for pain, how much residual bleeding to expect, and when she should call her doctor.

The woman sat up as the intern brought in the wheelchair. It wasn't until we were helping her off the table that I realized I was still holding her hand. She and I looked at each other. "Everything's going to be okay," I said.

Her eyes looked sad and tired, but no longer scared. "Thanks," she said. We let go of each other's hands and the intern wheeled her back to the room she had been in before, to rest until the anesthetic wore off.

I stayed behind to help clean up. The senior and I assembled the used instruments to be cleaned and gathered up the sheets to put into the laundry. As we worked, the senior reviewed the D & C with me, going over techniques and parts of it that I had been unable to see. "By the way," she said, "thanks. You really did help." I smiled.

The intern came back into the room. "How did I do?" she asked the senior. "Great," said the senior. "You did a nice job."

"Thanks for taking me through it," said the intern, smiling. She started helping us clean up. Her movements were quick, and she seemed happy. She looked at me. "Sorry to steal a procedure from you," she said. "Hopefully there will be another D and C before you finish your month here—I won't butt in, and you can do something on that one."

"Sure, thanks," I said, but it didn't matter so much to me anymore. I knew that there would always be something I could do.

MR. PARZIALE

*T*o us, subacute bacterial endocarditis meant a potentially life-threatening infection that ate away at the valves and lining of the heart.

To Mr. Parziale, it meant absolutely nothing.

*W*e tried to explain about bacteria and blood tests and blood cultures and findings on echocardiograms. He wouldn't listen.

"I am an old man," he would say. "I am supposed to be weak and tired. This is what happens to a body when it gets old."

But fevers aren't a normal part of aging, we would point out, saying that the fevers he had been having were a sign that there was an infection in his body.

"So I have an infection," he would say. "So give me some pills to take."

Not for this infection, we told him. The treatment for this

infection is six weeks of intravenous antibiotics, in the hospital.

This was utterly preposterous to him. "Absolutely not," he said firmly. "I have things to do."

Mr. Parziale was seventy-eight years old. He'd been born in Italy and emigrated to Boston as a young man. He had built a business, a small but successful grocery store that he still managed with the help of his two sons.

He told us again and again that there was nothing wrong with him and certainly nothing wrong with his heart. He insisted that he had never been sick.

"Every day, I have been at my store," he said. "Ask anybody."

When we asked more detailed questions, he did admit that he'd had rheumatic fever as a child. But when we tried to explain how the rheumatic fever had left one of his heart valves damaged and thus more susceptible to infection, he looked at us as though we were crazy to suggest that an illness he'd had when he was nine years old could have anything to do with his health at seventy-eight. Also, the whole concept of the heart as a structure with chambers and valves and a lining was something he seemed unable to understand.

He sat on the chair in the room at Massachusetts General Hospital, dressed in his street clothes. His sons stood next to him. We, the medical team, filled up most of the rest of the room; there was the attending, the junior, three interns, and two medical students doing their internal medicine clerkship, including me. We must have been intimidating, with our white coats, identification badges, and stethoscopes, but Mr. Parziale was not easily intimidated.

"Absolutely not," he said.

His sons pleaded with him. They said that if he wouldn't think about himself, he should think about them and their mother and all the other people who loved him and needed him around.

When they mentioned their mother, he seemed to listen. He said he couldn't leave the store; they said they could manage without him. He frowned; they quickly said they could manage for a little while.

"I will try it," he said finally. "But I am only trying it. And I am not staying for six weeks."

Doctors have a simple approach to thinking about patients and illness. They look at the symptoms, the findings on physical exam, and the results of laboratory tests, and they make a diagnosis. Once the diagnosis is made, the main and really only goal is to treat and try to eradicate the illness, in the most effective way possible. Once the diagnosis is made, the patient is often thought of only in terms of his or her illness. The doctors on the team didn't think of Mr. Parziale as a proud Italian businessman, the way they would have thought of him had they met him anywhere else but the hospital. They thought of him as the man with endocarditis.

The nurse gave Mr. Parziale a hospital gown to put on, but he said he didn't wear dresses, and he ended up tucking it into his pants like a shirt. I put in his IV. He said it didn't hurt, but he flinched when the needle entered his skin and grew very pale when his blood flowed back through the catheter.

The other patient in Mr. Parziale's room was an eighty-six-year-old man who had suffered a bad stroke. He was very disoriented and would randomly shout out unintelligible words, often at night. He was also frequently incontinent, and although the nurses were quick to clean him up, the room often smelled of urine or feces. Mr. Parziale kept the curtain between the two beds drawn and never said anything about the shouting or the smell. He was a very polite man.

He did try for a few days. He put up with being awakened at odd hours to have his vital signs and IV checked. He tolerated the frequent and unscheduled visits from us, the bad food, the lack of privacy, even the blood tests, although the sight of his blood continued to make him very pale. His wife brought in some pajamas, and we let him wear those instead of the hospital gowns.

He did try, but by the end of the week he became unpleasant and surly and refused to be examined. His sons came to us, asking if there was any other way of treating this infection, because their father was threatening to leave. We told them no.

The first time he tried to leave, the nurse caught him and called the security guards. The second time he was smarter; he waited until the nurses' change of shift, when they were busy, and slipped out. Both times he ripped out his IV, and both times he bled for quite a while. We saw the blood on the sheets. It probably didn't hurt much, but it must have been horrible for him to watch himself bleed.

The doctors on the team rolled their eyes and shook their heads when they talked about Mr. Parziale's escape attempts. He just doesn't understand, they all said. As I listened, I couldn't help wondering if we were the ones who didn't understand.

His sons brought him back to the hospital the next day. They literally carried him into the emergency room and refused to let him leave. They took shifts at his room on the ward after he was admitted, to make sure he stayed, and made arrangements with the nurses and security guards when they couldn't be there. I put lots of extra tape on his IV.

Mr. Parziale stopped speaking to his sons. He would not speak to anyone, not even his wife. He would not watch television or read the books and magazines they brought; he just stared out the window in stony, silent protest. He would eat, but only a few bites; he never finished a meal. He allowed the vital signs examinations, but he never made eye contact or moved more than was absolutely necessary.

After about two weeks, Mr. Parziale began to change. He began to watch television and to answer questions in a muted monotone. He got up and walked the hall when the nurse told him he had to exercise. He even put on a hospital gown. It was as if his silent protest gradually melted into silent defeat.

I don't think it was that he decided we were right, because he never did understand what endocarditis was. I don't think he decided to be cooperative for the sake of his family, either, because he barely spoke to them or even looked at them when they came to visit.

His sons were relieved because they didn't have to do shifts anymore, but his wife was worried. She watched her husband's sluggish movements with an anxious look on her face. His hair became unkempt and his face unshaven. His eyes were dull, and it seemed to me that he suddenly looked very old.

I kept telling myself that without this treatment, Mr. Parziale's illness would most likely kill him eventually. We are being responsible, I told myself; we are doing what's best for him.

He stayed in the hospital the full six weeks, without attempting to leave again. The blood tests and the echocardiograms showed remarkable improvement. He has done well, we said to each other on rounds. He is very lucky. Yet as I looked at his dull eyes and slumped shoulders every day when we went in to see him, I felt uneasy and confused.

If a patient has a concept of himself and his illness that is entirely different from ours, doesn't this change our responsibility somehow? When our treatments rob a patient of his pride and self-worth, doesn't this affect what is best for him? I kept thinking that we should have done something differently. Maybe if we had listened to him some more and tried to understand him better, maybe if we had tried to find some way to share our power with him—maybe that would have made a difference.

The day Mr. Parziale left the hospital, he smiled politely and thanked the nurses, although he didn't say what he was thanking them for. His shirt and pants hung on him; he'd lost a lot of weight during his hospital stay. I watched him walk down the hall on his wife's arm. His feet dragged, and he didn't respond to her animated, although forced, chatter.

His endocarditis is cured, I thought, but he is still ill. We replaced one illness with another.

ONE NIGHT

ON

OBSTETRICS

*T*he woman was very quiet as she lay on the bed in the labor room. Sweat glistened on her forehead, and her straight brown hair was tangled and pressed against her head. As another contraction began she closed her eyes and stiffened. Her husband offered his hand, but she held the side rail of the bed instead, her knuckles whitening as she clenched.

Her husband looked up at Rick, the obstetrical resident. "Can't you give more terbutaline? The contractions seem to be worse."

"We're doing everything we can, Mr. Kelley," said Rick.

Mr. Kelley looked over at his wife. He put his hand on her shoulder. "I know you are, I'm sorry," he said. "It's just that I can't believe this is happening again."

Mrs. Kelley opened her eyes as the contraction passed. "It hasn't happened yet," she snapped.

"Honey, things don't look good."

"I don't care. I'm not giving up yet."

I wished I were standing closer to the door so that I could slip out; I felt uncomfortable being there.

"The cerclage is still in place," said Rick. "We can keep it there if we can stop her labor. We are giving all the medicine we can—we'll just have to wait and see what happens. I'll check back in a little while."

I followed Rick out of the room. As soon as we were out of earshot, he said, "Her husband's right. Things don't look good."

Mrs. Kelley had been pregnant four other times, and each pregnancy had ended in miscarriage. This time she had come to one of the Brigham and Women's Hospital obstetricians who specialized in high-risk pregnancies to see if anything could be done. He felt that part of the problem could be that her cervix was incompetent, that it gave way too soon and couldn't hold a baby inside. So he did a cerclage, tying the cervix closed. That seemed to help; she had gone farther with this pregnancy than she had with any of the others. But now she was in premature labor, and if it could not be stopped, there would be no choice but to untie the cerclage and let the baby be born. She was twenty-two weeks pregnant, just two weeks shy of what the pediatricians could save. At twenty-four weeks the baby had a chance, albeit slim. At twenty-two weeks it would certainly die.

Labor and Delivery was full of motion and noise. Doctors and nurses gathered at the curved charting area in the middle of the room, writing progress notes, making phone calls, talking to one another. Arranged around the periphery were the labor rooms.

It was my first shift on call during my obstetrics rotation, a rotation required during the third year. I was overwhelmed by everything around me.

I sat down on the only unoccupied chair. Every once in a while I heard a woman crying out in pain, sometimes even screaming. Suddenly the crying or screaming would stop, there would be a short stillness, and then you'd hear the cry of a baby. Over and over again, it was the same. There was something about the combination of sounds that was unreal and wonderful. The mood of the unit was an odd mixture of tension, practiced calm, and joy. Everyone working there had attended birth after birth, but each one had its own possibility of something unexpected. Here it was a little different from most hospitals, because Brigham and Women's was a high-risk obstetrical referral center. Although most of the labor rooms were occupied by women who had nice normal uncomplicated pregnancies, some held women who had real problems, women like Mrs. Kelley. It added an extra dimension to the tension, and it made everyone more careful.

Rick leaned against the counter above the desk, writing on Mrs. Kelley's chart. He was dressed in the usual blue scrubs with a white coat over them. His light brown hair was mussed from putting on and taking off the paper bouffant caps everyone had to wear in the delivery rooms along the back hall. Those rooms were big, sterile, and full of supplies and could be used as operating rooms. Women were taken there for cesarean sections or complicated deliveries where extra equipment and people were needed. Rick had been spending a lot of time in those rooms that day.

"Do you have any questions about anything?" he said to me. I loved his accent; he was from Alabama, and even the most ordinary sentences sounded musical when he spoke them.

"No, you've explained everything really well," I said. I felt bad for him. The last thing he probably wanted right then was to be saddled with a medical student to supervise and teach, especially one who was brand new. He had ignored me a bit, if only to get his work done, but he had tried to include me on interesting patients and bring me to deliveries.

Donna, the nurse who was taking care of Mrs. Kelley, came up to Rick. She was one of the older nurses, with short graying black hair. She leaned on the counter, her face serious. "We aren't getting anywhere," she said. "Her contractions are more frequent now, and stronger. I hate to say it, but I think that cerclage is going to have to come out."

Rick was quiet; his shoulders fell. "Yeah," he said finally. "I can't think of anything else we could try. Let me page McGuire." Dr. McGuire was the high-risk obstetrician who had been following Mrs. Kelley. He had come in to the hospital from home when Mrs. Kelley called to say she was in labor. While we were waiting to see if the medicines would work, he had been checking on some of his patients in the hospital. Rick picked up the phone to page him, and Donna went back into Mrs. Kelley's room.

I watched her as she went. My chair had wheels on it; by pushing myself backward a few feet, I could get a clear view into the room. Mrs. Kelley was lying stiffly, staring up at the ceiling; tears were running down her cheeks. Mr. Kelley sat slumped over on the chair beside the bed, his face in his hands. He seemed to be crying, too. I sat there and watched, feeling as though I were in the room with them. I knew I should stop watching, but their sadness held me.

Rick hung up the phone. "McGuire agrees—cerclage has got to come out. He'll be down in a minute. I'm sure he'd let you watch if you'd like."

I pulled my chair back to where it had been so that I couldn't see into the room anymore. "No, thanks," I said.

Dr. McGuire arrived quickly. He was small and grayhaired, dressed in scrubs like Rick. He nodded to Rick, and they went into Mrs. Kelley's room.

I had known that things went wrong with deliveries sometimes. I knew that sometimes babies were stillborn, or that women sometimes died in childbirth. But I had thought that modern medicine had made such things rare, and I had certainly not expected to encounter something like this so soon. Suddenly birth seemed so dangerous, so tenuous.

I wandered around Labor and Delivery for a while, listening to the noises and reading the charts of the ward patients. When I went back near Mrs. Kelley's room I could hear Rick's and Dr. McGuire's voices, but I couldn't make out what they were saying. Donna was talking, too, in soothing, soft tones. Mrs. Kelley was moaning. The moans grew louder and then stopped. There was a silence and then some more soft voices. Finally Donna came out, wheeling a bassinet. She wheeled it into one of the empty rooms; I followed.

Donna turned on some warming lights and pulled them over so they shone over the bassinet. "There's not much point in keeping her warm, I guess," she said. "But until the pediatricians come and give the final word, I feel better with the lights on her."

It was a tiny little girl. Her skin was pale and translucent, her eyes tightly shut, and she had faint light hair. She wasn't breathing, but her heart was beating; I could see it as a flutter under the thin wall of her chest.

"Mrs. Kelley didn't want to keep her with her?" I asked.

"Mrs. Kelley said her good-byes," said Donna. "She said she didn't want to watch her daughter die."

The pediatric resident came into the room. He was dressed in scrubs, a half-tied mask around his neck. He carried a box with him, filled with equipment for the resuscitation of newborns.

"This the twenty-two-weeker you called us about?" he asked, looking down at the baby.

"Yeah," said Donna.

"Sure of the dates?"

"Yeah. If anything, could be more like twenty or twenty-one weeks."

"Looks it. So what do you want me to do?"

"Oh, I don't know," said Donna. "Take a look at it, tell us there's nothing anybody can do, so we can tell the mother that's what the pediatrician said, too."

Mother. Mrs. Kelley was a mother, of a baby that was going to die, that was really already dead except that her heart was beating. It would stop soon. You need to be able to breathe to live, and this little girl didn't have enough lungs to breathe.

The pediatrician took the stethoscope from around his neck and listened to the baby's chest. He ran his fingers over her skin, examining her.

"This baby never had a chance," he said finally. "She does look more like twenty weeks or so. If she had stayed in just a little longer . . ."

"Yeah, I know," Donna said a little abruptly. "Thanks for coming by." She left the room. The pediatrician put his stethoscope back around his neck, sighed, and left, too.

I stayed to look at the baby a little longer. She was a fetus, not really a baby, but you could imagine the baby she would have become. I looked at her tiny nose, touched her tiny hand. They would have loved you so much, I thought. I could feel myself starting to cry, so I left the room. I wished there were someone to hold her until her heart stopped beating; she looked so alone. I didn't know if they would let me, but even if they would have, I didn't think I could do it.

I don't know how long it was before the baby's heart stopped beating; I avoided the room. I know that an hour or so later the room was empty and Mrs. Kelley had been moved upstairs.

Rick and I didn't talk much for the next couple of hours. He was morose and brusque. He finally asked one of the other obstetricians who was there if I could go to a normal delivery with her; I wasn't sure if he was trying to cheer me up or whether he just wanted to be left alone. The patient, who seemed relaxed despite her pain, was a woman in her mid-thirties having her fourth child. I stood by and watched as the obstetrician gently held the head of the baby as it emerged, suctioned out the mouth, guided the baby's shoulders under the pelvic brim, and then deftly caught the baby as it came slithering out.

"It's a girl!" she said, and held her up for the mother, who smiled an exhausted but radiant smile. The baby screamed, and we all smiled—the doctor, the nurse, the parents, and I. The doctor put clamps across the umbilical cord in two places and gave the father a pair of big scissors to cut the cord in between the clamps. The nurse took the baby and dried her off. The baby screamed and screamed. The screams were loud and vigorous and wonderful. The nurse swaddled her in a blanket; contained again, the baby quieted. The nurse brought her to the parents, who held her together and kissed.

I slipped out, feeling immensely happier. Not seeing Rick anywhere, I found a chair, sat down, and flipped through an obstetrical journal that was lying in the nurses' station. There were fewer people around than earlier; there weren't very many patients, and since it was almost two in the morning the staff consisted only of people who absolutely had to be there.

Suddenly there was a commotion outside Labor and Delivery: a girl was screaming, and there were other voices, too. The doors swung open, and two ambulance attendants wheeled in a very pregnant young blond girl. Behind them was the Labor and Delivery charge nurse, who looked angry, and an older woman in a worn, frayed coat who looked scared.

"Where do we put her?" one of the ambulance attendants said loudly, looking around him. The girl on the stretcher was still screaming.

"What do you think you're doing?" said the charge nurse in a controlled terse voice, as she put herself between the stretcher and the rest of Labor and Delivery. "You can't just barge in here."

"Look, lady, what do you want me to do?" yelled the attendant above the girl's screams. "They sent us here from the emergency room. You want me to leave this screaming pregnant woman out there in the hallway?"

The charge nurse opened her mouth to say something and then shut it. "Okay," she said. She pointed to her right. "Room seventeen. Over there."

I followed them over. The older woman trailed behind. She looked to be in her late fifties, but it was hard to tell. The charge nurse came up to her. "Who are you?" she asked.

"I'm her mother," she said.

"Great," said the charge nurse. "Could you answer a few questions?" The woman nodded. I stayed to listen.

The girl's name was Janie Peters, and she was nineteen years old. Her mother didn't know when her due date was, but she thought it was sometime soon. It was Janie's third pregnancy; she'd had an abortion when she was fifteen, and she had a two-year-old daughter. Her mother said she didn't know if there had been any problems with this pregnancy, but she didn't think so.

The charge nurse asked who Janie's doctor was. Janie's mother said she didn't have one.

"She kept meaning to make an appointment," she said sheepishly. "But she's been fine, really."

The charge nurse and I looked at each other. The charge nurse took a deep breath. "Okay," she said. "So what happened today?"

"I don't know," said Janie's mother. "She was fine, then all of a sudden she started saying that her stomach was killing her. At first I thought it was just labor, but something didn't seem right, so I called the ambulance."

I couldn't read the charge nurse's face. She wrote a few things down on a piece of paper and told the mother to wait in the waiting room.

"Can't I be with her?"

"Let us get her settled first, okay? We'll come get you as soon as possible."

The girl was still screaming. The mother looked nervously into the room.

"We'll take care of her, don't worry," said the charge nurse.

The mother looked into the room again, then walked slowly to the swinging doors and out to the waiting room.

Rick came up to us. "What's up?" he asked the charge nurse, pointing to the room with the screaming girl.

"Nineteen-year-old, third pregnancy, at about term, no prenatal care, who just rolled in by ambulance with abdominal pain. Nancy's getting an IV and bloods and putting her on a monitor."

"Thanks," said Rick. He motioned me to follow him.

The girl lay on the stretcher, writhing, trying to curl up on her side, while Nancy, one of the nurses, was trying to put the monitor straps around her abdomen. She had put on a hospital gown, and an IV was in her left forearm.

"Please, do something," she was saying, more softly now than before. "Please, help me, this is killing me."

Nancy was still trying to get the monitor straps on. There were two of them—one to pick up contractions, the other to pick up the fetal heartbeat. "Try to calm down, Janie, and stop moving. We are going to help you, but we need to make sure everything is okay with you and the baby." She looked up. "Oh, good, Rick, you're here. She's been having bleeding—and look at that blood pressure."

Rick picked up the nursing flow sheet, and I looked over his shoulder. Blood pressure was 160/120: way too high. "Did you get a urine yet?" he asked.

Nancy looked up at Rick as she struggled with the straps. Her hair hung in front of her eyes; she had no free hand to push it out of the way. "No, Rick, I haven't gotten to that yet."

There is a condition that can occur during pregnancy called toxemia. Symptoms are high blood pressure, swelling of the hands or feet, and protein in the urine. It varies in its severity, but it can be dangerous, even life-threatening, to pregnant women and the babies they are carrying. It can cause major problems with the placenta, strokes, liver problems, and internal bleeding. Because it can be so serious, and because complications are often avoidable if it is detected early, it is screened for very carefully during prenatal visits. If Janie had never been to a doctor during this pregnancy, there was no telling how long she might have been suffering from toxemia and what damage it might have done.

Nancy finally had the straps around Janie's huge abdomen. She was staring at the monitor readings, frowning. She fiddled with the straps a little, moving the round plastic leads into slightly different places. She reached down to Janie's wrist, taking her pulse. She motioned for Rick to look at the monitor.

"I'm having trouble getting the baby's heart rate," she said. "All it seems to keep picking up is hers."

Rick looked at the monitor readings and asked the charge nurse to get the portable ultrasound.

"When did you last feel the baby move?" he asked Janie. His voice was calm but serious.

"I don't know," said Janie.

"Did you feel it today?"

"It hurt so much today, I don't know. Maybe yesterday."

Nancy kept moving the straps around, but the heart rate monitor kept reading ninety to a hundred. That's low for a baby's heart rate. It was also very regular; babies' heart rates usually go up and down with contractions and other stimuli. Nancy put her fingers on Janie's wrist in between adjustments. "It's still hers," she kept saying.

The charge nurse wheeled in the small portable ultrasound that was kept in Labor and Delivery. Nancy took off the monitor straps. Rick squeezed some gel onto Janie's belly and began to move the ultrasound probe across it. Janie watched him carefully. She was still obviously in pain, but she was quieter now, intent on what Rick was doing.

"Is something wrong?" she asked.

"We're just going to take a look," said Rick.

I looked over Rick's shoulder at the screen. The image was blurred, but I could make out shapes that looked like parts of a baby. Rick looked up at me. "There's the head, see?" he said, pointing to the image on the screen. He frowned.

"What?" I asked.

He looked at Janie and shook his head slightly. Not in front of her, he was telling me. I looked more closely at the image. The shape of the head looked a little funny; it didn't seem quite round. Then he moved the probe up and I could see the spine.

"What are you looking for?" I asked.

"The heart," he said.

He moved the probe around a little bit more, and the heart came into view, with its four chambers and valves. Something wasn't right, though. It took a few seconds, but suddenly I realized what was wrong: the heart wasn't beating.

The baby was dead.

I froze. Janie looked at me. "What's wrong with the baby?" she asked. "Is there something wrong with the baby?"

Rick moved the probe up to the placenta, his eyes fixed on the screen. "Could you get her mother?"

"Sure," I said, glad to escape.

Her mother was sitting in the waiting room, on the chair closest to the door. She held her coat and purse tightly in her lap. She stood up when she saw me. I told her the doctor wanted to talk to her and led her in, walking quickly so I wouldn't have to say anything else. When we got to the room, Rick had finished with the ultrasound and was wiping the gel off Janie's skin.

Mrs. Peters put her coat and purse on a chair in the corner and went over to Janie. She took her hand and kissed her on the forehead, and then she turned to Rick. "Tell us what's wrong," she said.

Rick took a step back and leaned against the wall. He seemed defeated, somehow. "I'm afraid the baby has died," he said.

Janie looked startled. She stared at Rick, wide-eyed and pale. "What do you mean?" asked Mrs. Peters.

"Just that. The baby's heart has stopped beating. I'm really sorry."

"But how? Why? Everything was fine," said Mrs. Peters, clutching Janie's hand.

"Everything wasn't fine, actually," said Rick. He explained about toxemia and told them that the placenta had torn away from the inside of the uterus. If the placenta wasn't attached, the baby couldn't survive. "It's called an abruption," he said. "That's why she's been having bleeding and so much pain."

"Can you take it out of her?" asked Mrs. Peters. "Can you make it stop hurting?"

"We can't take it out by a C-section, if that's what you

mean," said Rick. "It wouldn't be safe, and it could make future pregnancies more complicated. But we don't need to take it out—it's coming out on its own."

"You mean she's gonna go through labor like with a regular baby, only when the baby comes out it's gonna be dead?"

Rick nodded.

"No," Janie said. "Please. Take it out of me now."

She began to cry. Her mother caressed her face, wiping her tears.

"I can't," said Rick. "I don't think it's going to be very long, anyway. We'll give you medication to help the pain."

Janie wasn't listening. "Mama, my baby's dead," she was saying over and over again.

Rick was right; it wasn't very long. Less than two hours later he came to find me. "We're going down to the delivery room with Janie Peters. Come on."

I put on a cap, a mask, and shoe covers and followed Rick into Delivery Room Two.

Janie was on the table in the center of the room, her feet up in stirrups. The pain medication must have taken effect; although she looked uncomfortable, she was no longer writhing. The warming table where babies are put initially after they are born was draped with a blanket, but the warming lights weren't on. Nancy was busy assembling instruments and putting them on a small draped table near Janie's feet. She stopped what she was doing and went over to Janie.

"Janie," she said gently, "do you want to see the baby after it comes out?"

Janie was quiet for a few seconds. "No," she said finally. "Not if it's really dead."

It was a quick delivery. Rick laid the baby on the warming table. It was a boy, with lots of hair and long fingers. He was scrawny, more evidence that the placenta had been in trouble for a long time. He was very blue, and from the way his head had started to cave in on the sides, he had probably been dead for a couple of days. Nancy wrapped him up quickly, put him in a bassinet, and wheeled him away. I looked over at Janie, who suddenly looked worn and frail. She was shaking, and her eyes were red and wet.

She saw me looking at her, and motioned to me. I went over to her.

"What was it?" she asked. I knew what she meant, but I wanted desperately not to answer.

"Janie, I just need to put a few stitches in and then we'll get you back to your room," said Rick. "Claire, could you give me a hand until Nancy gets back?"

Quickly, gratefully, I moved down to the foot of the bed, put on sterile gloves, and handed Rick the things he needed. Janie didn't ask her question again.

I wanted to be angry at her, to yell at her that she might have been able to prevent her baby's death, but all I felt was sad. I tried to imagine what it must feel like to carry a baby for nine months, or five and a half months in Mrs. Kelley's case, to know it and feel it move and then to have it die. I wanted to be angry, but I couldn't; it was too horrible.

I was supposed to see patients in the obstetrical outpatient clinic the next day, but Rick sent me home after the early morning Labor and Delivery rounds.

"It was a rough night," he said. "You can go to clinic tomorrow. Go get some sleep."

I didn't argue; I wanted to go home. I thanked him, quickly changed out of scrubs into my jeans and sweater, grabbed my coat, and practically ran out of the hospital.

Outside, it was gray and wet. The cold winter wind blew right through my jeans. I pulled my coat closer around me and walked quickly down Brookline Avenue. Ahead of me at the intersection, a young woman was crossing the street with two small children, one in a stroller, the other holding her hand. They might not make it across the street before the light changes, I thought suddenly. The little boy is walking so slowly, why doesn't she pick him up? My heart beat faster, and I walked more quickly. I'll go and pick him up, I thought; then she can just push the stroller, and it won't take so long. The light changed as I reached the intersection. All the cars waited as she got the stroller onto the sidewalk and helped the little boy up onto the curb.

Doesn't she realize how fragile everything is? I wondered as the cars whizzed by me. Doesn't she realize how careful and grateful we have to be?

COACH

"**Y**ou've got to be careful with your breathing," he would tell me. "That's how to avoid stitches. If you get one, though, keep running. Slow down a little and try to breathe deeply, but keep running. If you stop and walk, it's not going to help, and you'll ruin your times."

"Okay, coach," I'd say.

As part of my internal medicine clerkship, every third night I stayed at the hospital with the residents. I helped out with whatever work needed to be done, and I wrote admission notes and orders on certain patients being admitted to the hospital. Unless they became very sick or their cases became complicated, I would follow these patients during their hospitalizations and help in their care. Mr. Bowman was one of "my patients," a sixty-seven-year-old man who had been diagnosed with colon cancer several years earlier. A large section of his colon had been removed, so large that it had been necessary to do a colostomy. Now, instead of passing through to his rectum, his stool came out through a hole in his abdominal wall into a plastic bag. He had been hospitalized because recently he had noticed some blood in the stool, and his doctor was worried there might be a recurrence of the cancer.

When I was taking his history, I asked him if he worked. No, he told me, he was retired.

"What did you do?" I asked.

"I coached track."

"Really? I'm a runner."

"You don't look like a runner."

"Why?" I asked. I was hurt; I ran upward of forty miles a week and had actually managed to finish the Boston Marathon the month before. I did Nautilus at the local gym whenever I had time, was careful about what I ate, and was proud of my leanness.

"Your earrings are too big."

I reached up and touched my earrings. They were dangly intertwined hoops that fell almost to my shoulders.

"I don't wear them when I run," I said.

*T*he initial round of tests showed nothing abnormal. "So far, this is very reassuring," said Dr. Jollens, his doctor, as we reviewed Mr. Bowman's chart together. I liked Dr. Jollens. He was younger than most of the attending physicians on the private service, and he was always happy to teach medical students.

"I guess the next thing to do is go take a look," he said.

"Endoscopy?" I asked. This meant taking a special instrument with a fiber-optic lens and inserting it into Mr. Bowman's colon, probably through the colostomy. By doing this, Dr. Jollens could look directly at the inside of the colon and see if there was anything that looked like cancer. He could also take a sample of any unusual tissue while he was in there.

"Yep," he said. "I'll check my schedule."

"Speedwork is very important," Mr. Bowman told me.

"But I don't like speedwork," I said. "I like to go out and just run."

"All the good long-distance runners do speedwork. Got a track near you?"

"Yes."

"Four laps to the mile?"

"I think so."

"Okay. Start with one fast lap to one slow, work up to three fast to one slow, for about five miles. At least once a week, better twice."

"I'll try."

He had his wife bring in his scrapbook to show me. There were newspaper clippings from the college paper and the local paper about his team's victories. There seemed to be a lot of victories, which I pointed out.

He smiled. "Why would I cut it out if we lost?"

There were pictures of him crossing the finish line of the Boston Marathon. Not first, but it looked as though he had done respectably. There was one from 1941, when he was twenty-one, and one next to it from 1947. He looked different in the second picture, somehow. He looked stronger and tougher and much, much older.

He noticed my pause. His eyes suddenly looked sad. "Between those two marathons, I went to war."

There were more marathon pictures. The last looked recent. "That's from 'eighty. Ran it the last time then, when I was sixty—right after my sixtieth birthday. Then I got sick, and they cut me open and stuck this thing on me." He pointed to the colostomy bag, which I could just make out under his shirt.

"I'm sorry," I said.

"No need to be sorry for me, young lady. I'm just fine." He took the scrapbook from me and closed it. He picked up the newspaper from his bedside table and stared at the front page.

"I guess I'll leave you alone, then," I said.

He didn't answer. I got up from the chair, picked up my stethoscope, and headed for the door.

"Be sure to do your speedwork," he said as I was almost out. I turned around. He smiled; it was a small and brief smile. I smiled back.

We didn't talk much about his condition, Mr. Bowman and I, nor did I touch him often. Whereas usually I examined my patients every day, with Mr. Bowman it was different. When he was first admitted I examined him, which was routine, but there was something about him that intimidated me, so my examination was relatively brief and modest. I knew the intern would do a more thorough physical. Lines were drawn early.

We were almost done with morning rounds, making our plans for the day, when the junior's beeper went off. He reached for a phone, called the operator, and answered the page.

"Great," he said. "Fine. I'll send her."

He hung up and turned to me. "That was Jollens. He's got Bowman in the endoscopy suite now, wants you to meet him there."

"But—but we're not done with rounds," I said.

"Close enough," said the junior. "We'll catch you up when you get back."

"But I'm supposed to present to the attending at ten."

"The other students can present. What's your problem, Claire? Don't you want to go? Jollens is trying to be nice and teach you something."

I was stuck. I tried to say something to sound grateful, and the junior sent me off.

Mr. Bowman was lying on the stretcher in the last room off the hallway in the endoscopy suite. Dr. Jollens was assembling the endoscope and its attachments. He motioned toward the stool next to him.

"Claire! Good, you're here. Have a seat."

I sat down tentatively on the edge of the stool. I nodded hello to Mr. Bowman, who nodded back. He didn't smile, and I immediately felt uncomfortable. He usually smiled when he saw me.

"Okay, all set. Time to get started. Ready, Jim?"

"I guess so," said Mr. Bowman.

Dr. Jollens pulled up the hospital shirt Mr. Bowman was wearing and pulled down the pants a little, so his abdomen was exposed. He took off the plastic bag around the stoma. I looked away, to be polite, as he inserted the endoscope into the colostomy. He looked into it intently.

"What a great view. Here, Claire, have a look."

I looked at Mr. Bowman, who was looking out the window. He turned his head, and I caught his eye. I raised my eyebrows, hoping he would understand my question, but he just looked at me blankly. I turned to Dr. Jollens.

"I don't want to make it take any longer, you know, by having me look, too."

"No problem. I put the teaching attachment on, so we can look at the same time. Here." He handed me the extra end of the scope and looked into his.

"What I'm looking at now is transverse colon."

I looked up at Mr. Bowman, who was watching me. I held up the end of the scope and raised my eyebrows again. This time he seemed to understand. I couldn't read his expression; I thought I saw a trace of a frown, but then he nodded slightly. I hesitated for a moment, then looked into the scope.

It was incredible. There was the inside of his colon, with its folds and creases and moist, colorful lining. I watched through my end of the scope as Dr. Jollens maneuvered to the beginning of the ascending colon, back through the transverse and then down along the descending colon. As he went along he talked about what we were seeing, explaining the structures and what cancer might look like. I had never seen anything like it before, and I was fascinated.

"You doing okay, Jim?" Dr. Jollens asked a few times.

"Sure, fine," Mr. Bowman would say, his voice tense. He seemed uncomfortable, but not in pain. I carefully kept my eyes on the scope; I didn't look up at him the whole time.

It was entirely normal. We didn't find anything that looked even remotely like cancer. Dr. Jollens took some biopsies anyway to send to the pathology laboratory, just to be sure, but he told Mr. Bowman he felt confident they wouldn't show anything worrisome.

Mr. Bowman and I didn't look at each other. I stared at a crack in the wall, and Mr. Bowman stared at Dr. Jollens.

"I should be getting back," I said as soon as Dr. Jollens stopped talking. "Thank you, Dr. Jollens. That was really interesting."

"Glad you could come over," he said as he packed up his endoscope.

Mr. Bowman was pulling up his hospital pants. "Thanks," I mumbled in his direction, and left quickly.

Mr. Bowman stayed in the hospital for two or three more days after that. Dr. Jollens wanted to run a few more tests, all of which failed to show anything. Mr. Bowman and I didn't talk much. He seemed a little cold toward me, and I felt awkward. I kept my visits brief and only asked how he felt and whether he had noticed any more blood in his stool; fine, he said, and no. A couple of times I started to say something else, about running or something in the news, but I stopped. The last night he was there I went in with Dr. Jollens and listened as Dr. Jollens told him that he didn't know exactly why he had blood in his stool, but it didn't seem to be anything serious, and there was no evidence of any cancer. They would do some more tests in a few months, to follow up, but in the meantime he shouldn't worry. Mr. Bowman thanked him and nodded to me without looking at me.

His wife came in to pick him up the next morning. Her gray hair was short and curly, and she wore a blue dress with big yellow flowers. She smiled at everyone as she walked down the hall, and she brought a freshly baked coffee cake for the nurses.

"I went to the deli yesterday and bought some of that salami you like," she told her husband as she packed the last of his belongings into his suitcase. "I'll fix us a nice lunch as soon as we get home."

I watched from the doorway. She looked up at me.

"Yes?"

"I'm—I'm the medical student. I just wanted to come say good-bye."

"Of course. You're the runner. Thank you so much for all your help."

"I didn't do anything, really."

Mr. Bowman was buttoning his sweater. He sat down on the edge of the bed and started to put on his shoes.

"Well, I'm sure you did. And you kept him company, which I certainly appreciate."

Mr. Bowman tied his shoelaces. He hadn't looked up.

"I liked talking with him," I said. I took a few steps into the room. "Really, I did. And he helped me with my running. He gave me some good advice."

Mr. Bowman looked up from his shoelaces.

"I did some speedwork like he—I mean you—told me to, yesterday. I've been doing the other stuff, too, like with my breathing and my stride and the way I hold my arms."

Mr. Bowman looked at me for a few seconds, and then he stood up. "Good," he said. He walked over to me. "Keep it up, and you'll knock at least a half hour off your marathon time next year."

I reached out my hand. "Maybe I'll see you out there?"

"You never know," he said, smiling, and took my hand. "Maybe."

TAKING CARE

OF

CHILDREN

*T*hree weeks old with fever, the triage nurse had written on the top of the nursing sheet. I looked at the vital signs: the temperature was 38.9 centigrade, about 102 degrees Fahrenheit. I picked up the nursing sheet and the other papers from the wooden box outside the exam room door. This was going to be a full septic workup—blood tests, bladder tap, spinal tap—and an admission to the hospital. It was going to be a first for me.

*M*y last course of medical school was an elective in pediatric emergency medicine at Children's Hospital, the hospital where I was going to do my residency. My main reason for taking the course was to get more experience working with children. Most of my medical school work had been with adult patients, and I was a little nervous about starting a residency in pediatrics.

Although I had written in my diary when I was twelve years old that I wanted to be a pediatrician, for the first couple of years of medical school I thought I would go into internal medicine instead. I thought it was more dignified and intellectual. By the end of my third-year clerkships, however, I realized that I liked pediatrics better. Pediatrics seemed like a more optimistic field, perhaps simply because children are more likely to get better than adults are. I liked the pediatricians better than the internists, too; I think the optimism wore off on them. They were a more casual and friendly bunch, and their humor was less black than the internists'.

Ultimately, though, what it boiled down to was that I liked children better than adults. I liked their simplicity, their wonder, their honesty. For them everything was, or could be, a game.

I knocked on the door and went in. Out of habit my eyes went first to the stretcher, but it was empty. A young African-American couple was sitting on two of the three chairs lined up against the wall; the other chair held a quilted diaper bag and a blue baby snowsuit, the kind that is really more of a bag than a suit. The woman was holding a sleeping baby wrapped in a white wool blanket. She and the man turned to look at me.

"Hi," I said. "I'm Claire McCarthy." I knew I should introduce myself as a medical student, but I found it hard to do. I thought that it started things out on the wrong foot. I preferred to tell people a little later, when I felt that I had gained at least a little of their confidence.

"I'm Jana Sanders," said the woman. "This is my husband."

The man just nodded at me. He sat forward with his arms crossed in front of him, his elbows leaning on his knees. His hair was very short, and he had a mustache. He wore wire-

rimmed glasses, and the way he stared at me, I thought he
was going to ask me for identification.

I looked at the papers. "And this is David," I said as
pleasantly as I could, looking down at the baby.

"Davy, actually," said Jana. "He's David junior, after my
husband, so we call him Davy." She was very soft-spoken,
although she might just have been nervous. She was a small
woman, round in the way most women are after giving birth.
Her hair was tightly braided in many rows and gathered
neatly at the nape of her neck. She wore a loose-fitting blue
corduroy dress that looked wrinkled and worn and had
probably doubled as a maternity dress. It contrasted sharply
with her husband's clothing: crisp khaki pants and an ex-
pensive-looking crew-neck sweater over a white button-
down shirt. His leather shoes looked newly polished. I tried
not to look at him; his stare was making me increasingly
uncomfortable.

I knelt down. "Hi, Davy," I said.

The baby stirred a little but didn't open his eyes. He made
some sucking noises, and his little hand came out from under the blanket. He reached out briefly into the air at nothing, perhaps stretching, and then he settled again, turning
his head slightly in toward his mother. He was a big baby,
with a lovely round head, lots of curly hair, and clear brown
skin.

"He's very handsome," I said.

"Thank you," said Jana, smiling. Her husband nodded
and seemed to soften his stare a little.

I sat on the edge of the small counter built into the wall,
pulled out my pen, and started asking the usual questions.
Jana answered hesitantly but completely, looking frequently
at her husband as if hoping that maybe he'd talk so she
wouldn't have to. Davy was her first baby, and she'd had a
normal pregnancy and a normal vaginal delivery without any

problems three days after her due date. She'd gone home after the usual two days, and the baby had been just fine. She was breast-feeding, and he fed well, as far as she could tell—at least he fed frequently and sucked for a long time and didn't seem hungry afterward, so she figured that meant he fed well. Everything had been fine until the night before. He'd been a little congested over the past few days, but that night he'd seemed much more congested, and he'd cried a lot and wouldn't sleep and wasn't sucking as well or as long as usual. In the morning she'd taken his temperature and found that he had a fever. She'd called the pediatrician, who had told her to bring him to the hospital.

"Has either of you or anyone else in the house been sick recently?" I asked.

"I have a cold," said Jana. "My husband had it last week, and then I got it." She looked up at me anxiously. "It's not a bad cold or anything," she said.

"It's okay," I said, but she still looked anxious.

I asked her to bring him over to the stretcher so I could examine him. She did so reluctantly and then stood close by. Her husband stood up, too, and stood next to her, looking down at the baby.

He was still asleep. I unwrapped the blanket gently so as not to wake him. Underneath he was undressed down to his diaper, as the nurses always ask the parents to do. I watched him for a few seconds. He was sleeping peacefully but would move occasionally in a very normal way, which was a good sign. Very ill babies tend to be either very irritable or very lethargic, and he clearly was neither. He was breathing comfortably, too. He did seem congested, as Jana had said, but it didn't seem to be troubling him very much. I felt the soft spot on the top of his head; it was nice and flat, not bulging the way it could be if there was meningitis or sunken as in dehydration. Carefully I examined his skin, looking for rashes that might offer a clue to the cause of his fever; there were none. I took my stethoscope off my shoulder and warmed its diaphragm in my hands for a few seconds before putting it on his chest. It was an adult stethoscope, and it looked huge against his small chest. His heart was beating at a normal rate, and he didn't have a murmur. When I listened to his breath sounds I could hear the congestion, but it was all from his nose; the lungs themselves were clear. He woke up and started to whimper when I pressed on his belly. His big eyes looked almost annoyed. I checked his mouth and ears; they were normal. His muscle tone and reflexes were fine. Besides the stuffy nose, he seemed well.

Now that he was fully awake, his whimper turned into a loud cry. I wrapped him back up in the blanket and gave him to Jana, who had been leaning over closer and closer, ready to snatch him up. She sat down, rocking and shushing him.

"So what do you think?" asked the father. His voice was deep and melodious, like the voice of a singer, but it had a stern edge.

"I think he probably just has a cold," I said.

Jana looked up at me and then at her husband. "I'm sorry," she said.

"Don't be sorry," I said. "There's nothing you could have done, and he's going to be fine."

"So if it's just a cold, then we can just go home, right?" asked the father.

I leaned against the counter. "Actually, no," I said. I explained how studies had been done that showed that although most of the time when babies had a fever it was just a virus and not something to worry about, sometimes it meant that there was a bacterial infection somewhere we couldn't see, like in the blood or the urine or the spinal fluid. The studies suggested that the safest thing to do with the really little babies, especially those less than a month old who would have trouble fighting such an infection, was to take samples of blood and urine and spinal fluid for culture and then bring the baby into the hospital for forty-eight hours of antibiotics and observation while we waited for the results of the cultures. If they were negative, which they usually were, the baby could go home.

So that's what we'd be doing with Davy, I told them. I said that Jana could stay with the baby the whole time if she wanted and continue breast-feeding. She just held the baby and stared at me. She looked as though she were going to cry but wanted to wait until I was out of the room. I told them that we had a special room for doing the tests, with all the equipment we needed and bright lights, and that I'd come to get the baby as soon as it was ready.

"Who does the tests?" the father asked.

"I do."

"Are you good at it?"

"Yes," I said without missing a beat, and felt a stab of guilt. Well, what was I supposed to say? Since the rotation had started I'd done all the components of a septic workup separately with one of the doctors supervising, and I'd done fine. I'd just never done a complete one by myself. That didn't mean I was bad at it, did it?

"I'm a fourth-year medical student," I said in an attempt at half honesty, "but I know what to do."

He didn't look pleased, but Davy started to cry and then Jana started to cry, so he was distracted, and I ducked out of the room.

I went to the charting area to talk to the senior resident, who was on the phone arranging an admission. When she got off, I told her about Davy and what I thought and what I was going to do. She didn't say much; it was a straight-forward protocol, and there wasn't much to say. She wrote down his name, medical record number, and pediatrician in the admission book.

"Are you okay doing a septic workup?" she asked.

"I think so," I said. "I've done all the parts, and I've watched them. It's my first full one alone, but I think I'll be okay."

Her phone rang again. "All right," she said. "Just let me know if you need help, and I'll come in."

I went to the treatment room to set everything up. It was a big room, three or four times as large as the exam rooms, with an adjustable stretcher in the middle. The far wall had attachments and tubing and everything needed for oxygen and suction and a cardiac monitor. The other walls were lined with medical supplies, and there was a big sink in the corner. The overhead lights were big and bright, and two big flexible round lamps, the kind they have in operating rooms, hung over the stretcher.

I laid out the needles and syringes and tubes and bottles I would need to collect the blood and spinal fluid and urine. I put out the alcohol and the Betadine and ripped pieces of cloth tape to fasten the IV to Davy's skin once I'd put it in a vein. I got a bag of IV fluid and attached some tubing and hung it on the hook over the stretcher. I laid it all out methodically and slowly in the order I'd need it. I reached up and turned on the lamps, adjusting them so they shone down on the stretcher. I sat down on the stool by the stretcher, looked at everything, and ran through all the procedures in my head.

This septic workup is important, I told myself, looking at the needles nervously. They suddenly looked very big and sharp. We need to know what's going on with Davy. He may seem like he just has a cold, but maybe the fever is from something else. We need to protect him, we need to take the best care of him we can.

I needed someone to hold the baby while I did the procedures, so I went looking for one of the aides. I found Ada, an older Puerto Rican woman who had been working in the emergency room for years and whom I liked very much. She was good with the children, she gave good advice about which vein to pick to draw blood from or put an IV into, and she was helping me with my Spanish.

"One meenute," she said. "I finish something first. I meet you there."

I went to get Davy. Jana had stopped crying; she looked resigned as she held her son, who had gone back to sleep. Her husband looked uncomfortable and restless. He was pacing back and forth in the tiny exam room.

"I'm all set," I said.

"Should we come?" asked Jana.

I didn't want them to, because it would make me nervous to have them watch, but they had a right to come, and I didn't want to be rude.

"You can if you want to, but you certainly don't have to. You won't be able to hold him while we do the tests. Some parents find it hard to watch." I wondered if I should have said that. "We'll bring him back as soon as we're done. It should take about twenty minutes, maybe a little longer."

Jana looked at her husband, who shrugged.

"You guys look really worn out," I said, trying another tactic. "Why don't you go get some coffee? We'll take good care of Davy."

The husband reached over and put his hand on Jana's shoulder. "Why don't we get some coffee, hon. I could use some."

Jana sighed. "I guess I don't really want to watch."

I felt a guilty relief.

She looked down at the baby and then up at me. "Can you carry him okay?"

"Oh, don't worry about that," I said. "I'm a veteran."

"You have children?"

I blushed. "No," I said. "I meant a veteran baby-sitter."

"Oh, I see," she said. "I guess that's almost the same."

It wasn't, of course, and I felt silly. I reached down, and she handed Davy to me gingerly. I took him, laid him down on the stretcher, wrapped his blanket around him snugly in the way I'd learned to do so that it wouldn't come undone, and with a little more confidence picked him back up again.

"Don't want him to get cold," I said, and smiled.

Jana smiled, too, and relaxed a little. She stood up and reached for her purse. "Okay, then," she said. "We'll be right back."

"Take your time," I said. "Everything will be fine."

They left the room, and I went out after them. Davy had woken up and was looking at me. He had beautiful eyes and a tiny, perfect nose. I cradled him in my arms and smiled at him as I walked down the hall. He seemed fascinated by my face.

Ada wasn't there yet when I got to the treatment room, so I put the baby on the stretcher. I pulled the stool closer and sat down. Davy stared up at the bright lights and started to whimper a little. I picked him up again and rested him on my knees.

"It's okay, sweetheart," I said to him softly in a singsong voice. "You're okay." I stroked the side of his cheek and played with his hand, which had worked its way out from under the blanket. I swayed my knees slowly back and forth. He seemed to like that and stopped whimpering.

I brought my face down close so he could see me better and smiled at him, still playing with his hand. He looked at me intently for a while and then smiled, too. I laughed.

Ada came into the room. She startled me, and I quickly put the baby back on the stretcher, embarrassed. Ada took over wordlessly in the natural way she always did. She picked him up, unwrapped him, and moved him higher up on the stretcher. I watched her and felt wistful and unsure.

"*Qué guapo,*" she said. ("What a handsome one.") She leaned forward with her elbows on the stretcher, her hands caressing the baby, waiting for me to get started.

"I'll do the bladder tap first," I said, although I didn't need to say it. Ada had been at many more septic workups than I and knew the routine much better than I did. A bladder tap is when a needle is inserted through the carefully cleaned abdominal wall into the bladder to collect urine. It's considered the "cleanest" way to get urine for culture, especially with uncircumcised baby boys like Davy.

Ada took down his diaper, and I cleaned the skin above his pelvis with Betadine and alcohol. He squirmed a little with the alcohol, which feels cold, but he didn't cry. He looked at me and then at the bright lights. I put on sterile gloves, picked up my needle and syringe, and felt for the top of his pelvis with the index finger of my left hand. Then I took a deep breath, lifted the needle, and stabbed it straight down into his lower abdomen.

Davy's eyes flew wide open, and he screamed so loudly that it frightened me. My first instinct was to pull the needle back out so I could stop hurting him immediately, but there was no urine in the syringe yet. I need to get the urine, I told myself and forced my hand to stay steady. I drew back on the syringe as I pushed the needle in a little farther, and bright yellow urine quickly started to fill it. I was relieved and anxious; it seemed to be filling so slowly, and I wanted so much to take that needle out. As soon as the syringe was about half-full I pulled it out and put a gauze pad on the needle hole. Ada pressed on the pad to stop any bleeding.

Davy was still screaming, and my hands shook as I recapped the needle, put aside the syringe, and cleaned up the

Betadine and alcohol. It was so violent to stab a needle into a baby's belly, and I couldn't believe I'd just done it. I'd done it once before with the senior resident; it hadn't seemed so violent then. I guess I'd been concentrating so hard on doing it right the first time that I hadn't thought about it.

Ada put a Band-Aid on the needle hole and picked Davy up. She rocked him in her arms, singing one of the Puerto Rican lullabies she sang to the children to comfort them. He stopped crying and looked up at her. Let me put him on my knees, I wanted to say. He likes that.

Ada looked up at me with a glance that clearly told me to get on with things. I took the sterile cloth off the spinal tap tray, put on a mask and a new pair of sterile gloves. She laid Davy back down on the stretcher; immediately he started to cry. She laid him on his side facing away from me, curled him up in a fetal position, and held him that way.

He kept crying. I carefully cleaned his back, concentrating very intently on exactly where I should put the needle. I stood up straight and tried to relax my shoulders. I took the sterile cloths, folded them carefully in triangles, and laid them across and over the baby so that only a diamond-shaped area of the back was exposed. This is my work area, I told myself. This is all of the baby I will allow myself to think about right now.

I picked up the spinal needle. Now I will think only about the procedure, I told myself. The needle is to enter one of the lower lumbar interspaces at an angle, pointing up toward the umbilicus. When the resistance stops and you feel the needle pop into place, the stylet should be removed to see if spinal fluid comes back. I did it carefully and delicately.

There was spinal fluid, and it was clear. This was a good sign; in meningitis, the fluid is usually cloudy. "I'm in," I said to Ada, who nodded and kept singing her lullabies. I got out the tubes and let the fluid drip into them. It dripped slowly, like water from a leaky faucet.

Jana's face flashed into my mind.

Quickly I started thinking about the talk we had been given on the risks of bacterial infection in babies with fevers, trying to remember the exact statistics. I couldn't remember. So I thought instead about the antibiotics I would need to write orders for when I was done with the septic workup. Three weeks old, let's see, that means ampicillin and gentamicin. I calculated the dosages in my head, based on Davy's weight, as the spinal fluid went drip, drip, into the four plastic tubes.

It was like drawing the world in, making it smaller, a category, an envelope into which only certain thoughts and emotions would fit.

When the tubes were filled I took out the needle and put the gauze on the needle hole for Ada to press again.

I was calmer now. I took off the mask and brought over the things I needed for drawing blood as Ada put a Band-Aid on Davy's spine. She laid him on his back. I looked only at his arm as I tied the tourniquet above his elbow and started probing with my index finger in the inside of his elbow, trying to find a vein. They are hard to see, but not so hard to feel if you know how. With a tourniquet they are raised and bounce back slightly when you press on them.

I thought I felt one, so I cleaned the skin with Betadine and alcohol. Ada held the arm steady for me, and I put the needle where I thought I felt the vein. Blood went into the tubing and syringe. Ada nodded approvingly. I felt happy. I don't think I even noticed if Davy was crying or not.

I portioned out the blood into the blood culture bottles and the tubes for the other tests. This was actually going very well. It was somewhat unusual to get everything in a septic workup on "the first stick"; usually it took at least a couple of tries, especially on the blood drawing. I was proud.

I felt a rush of confidence and briefly envisioned myself as one of the best interns, able to handle any procedure, any emergency. I saw myself in scrubs in the middle of the night moving from patient to patient, assessing each problem, taking care of it, and moving on to the next.

There was only the IV left to do. Ada was looking for a vein on Davy's hands.

"There," she said, pointing to a bluish line on the back of his right hand. It was a good vein, large for a baby and straight enough to slide the IV catheter into it easily.

I put the tourniquet on above his right wrist. He'd been quiet, but right then Davy started to cry.

"This will be quick," I told Davy, Ada, and myself. "We'll just put this IV in and then we'll be all done."

I cleaned the hand and took the catheter-covered needle out of its package. I held the hand, putting tension on the skin to hold the vein steady, and slid the needle into the skin in the direction of the bluish line.

Nothing happened. No blood return. Davy started to scream. I pushed the needle in farther. Davy screamed louder, and still nothing happened. I pushed it in a little farther, but I wasn't really concentrating on what I was doing. A tiny bit of blood came back, but at the same time I saw the blue line swell.

Ada shook her head. "Blown," she said. The needle had gone through the vein.

I didn't say anything. I took off the tourniquet, took out the needle, and put pressure on the hand with a gauze pad. Ada took his hand from me. She kept the pressure on the gauze and picked him up.

"*Ay, tranquilo, mi cielo,*" she said, putting him up on her shoulder, but he was inconsolable.

Let me hold him, I wanted to say. I'm the one who has hurt him. The rush of confidence receded.

I turned away and got out another IV catheter. This child needs this IV. He needs his antibiotics. He needed this whole septic workup, to take care of him, to do the safest thing for his health. And whether I like it or not, it's my job now.

Ada and I found another vein on his other hand, and this time I got the catheter in without any trouble. "All done, all done," I found myself saying, although I'm not sure to whom I was talking. I taped up and covered the IV to protect it and attached the tubing and fluid.

I went to reach for him to pick him up, to take him back to Jana and her husband, but Ada scooped him up before my hands reached him, and I remembered that the aides usually brought the children back.

"What room?" she asked.

"Nineteen," I said.

As I watched her go with him, holding the IV bag above her head so that gravity would keep the fluid going into the vein, I felt empty and uneasy. I didn't know if I could get used to this way of caring for children.

FACE

The EMTs brought him in still strapped into his car seat. One of them carried him in like a suitcase—there was something like a handle on top of the car seat—and put him down in the emergency room triage area. He and his family had been in a car accident, they told the nurse. The impact had been relatively minor, with little damage to the car or passengers. His parents had been taken to Brigham and Women's Hospital more as a precaution than anything else. His sister was entirely fine and had left the accident with a family friend. They brought the little boy to Children's emergency room just to be sure he wasn't hurt.

"Why'd you leave him in the car seat?" asked the triage nurse.

"Well, it was kind of an immobilizer," said one of the EMTs.

"Besides, just watch what happens when you try to take him out," said the other.

He was a little African-American boy who looked to be a little more than a year old. He wore a snowsuit with the hood up and tied tightly underneath his chin. His mittens were attached with little clasps to the sleeves of the snowsuit. He didn't appear hurt in any way, just scared; he watched the triage nurse carefully as she inspected his neck, arms, and legs, looking for any signs of trauma. There weren't any.

"Okay, big boy," she said. "Let's get you out of this thing."

She reached over to push the button that released the straps, and the little boy screamed. It was an angry scream and so loud that it startled all of us, except the EMTs.

"See?" said the one who had warned us. "I kinda figured it wasn't worth it. He looks fine."

The triage nurse reached for the straps again, and the little boy screamed again. This time it was bloodcurdling.

The triage nurse looked up at me. I kneeled down and checked everything she had checked.

"He does kind of look fine," I said. "I really don't think he's hurt."

"Are his parents coming soon?" the triage nurse asked the EMTs.

"They shouldn't be long. The father had some pain in his neck, and the mother hurt her arm, but it didn't look like it was fractured."

"Okay," said the nurse. "I'll take his vitals and then we'll just wait until they show up."

The little boy watched her closely but didn't protest as she untied his hood and pulled down the zipper of his snowsuit as far as she could. He tolerated having the stethoscope on his chest to count his heart rate and respiratory rate. He even let her take his blood pressure and sneak a thermometer in under his arm. As long as nobody tried to take him out of the car seat, he was fine.

Since nobody was with him, we couldn't put him in an exam room, so the triage nurse brought him in his car seat

to the charting area where the doctors and nurses were working and put him in the corner on the floor. One of the nurses
who was doing some paperwork pulled up a chair next to
him to keep an eye on him.

We all tried talking to him, but he just stared stonily at
us. I gave him a saltine cracker, which he held dutifully in
his hand but wouldn't eat. The nurse tried to give him some
juice from a cup; he looked at it as though he wanted some,
but he wouldn't drink. He watched everyone and everything
with his wide brown eyes. He looked frightened, but he
didn't move, and he didn't cry.

We tried distracting him. We brought brightly colored
stickers and tongue depressors and rings of keys, things that
children will usually grab for, but he just sat there clutching
the cracker, his face fiercely blank. We tried playing peeka-
boo, we tried making silly faces, but nothing worked. Nothing even got a reaction from him.

His parents arrived about forty minutes later, anxiously
asking for their son. His mother, a young woman dressed in
a suit, walked over quickly and knelt down in front of the
little boy.

"Oh, baby," she said, "are you okay?"

"He's fine," said the nurse who had been watching him,
"but he won't let us take him out of the car seat."

The little boy's eyes had grown even wider on seeing his
mother. He dropped the cracker on the floor and reached
his arms out toward her.

"Let's get you out of this, baby," said his mother, releasing
the straps.

As soon as the straps went over his head, the little boy
threw himself at his mother with all the force he could mus-
ter. She caught him and held him tightly to her. Then, all
of a sudden, the stony face dissolved, and he began to cry.
He buried his head in her chest and cried and cried.

FIRST
NIGHT

I wrote everything down on an index card as Paula, the senior resident of my team, told me how to manage diabetic ketoacidosis. We were sitting in a corner of the emergency room charting area, discussing my first admission as an intern.

It was the July after my graduation from medical school, and I had just started my residency in pediatrics. Although officially we were residents, those of us in the first year out of medical school were often called interns. It is a historical term; years ago all medical school graduates did an internship involving many areas of medicine prior to entering specialty training, or residency. For the most part now, that first year out is incorporated into residency, but the term *intern* has stuck. Part of the reason it has stuck is that interns are identifiably different from the other residents; especially at the beginning, they are obviously inexperienced, overwhelmed, and scared.

My first admission was a fifteen-year-old girl with diabetes who had stopped taking her insulin when her boyfriend broke up with her. Her mother found her barely conscious in the bedroom and called an ambulance. When she got to the emergency room she was in ketoacidosis, which is what happens to diabetics if they go too long without insulin. It can be life-threatening.

Fluids are the mainstay of therapy, Paula was telling me. FLUIDS, I wrote down.

"Approximate the deficit from your assessment of the clinical status of the patient," she said, "and calculate how much you need to give her to replace half of that over the first eight hours and the rest over the next sixteen. Plus, she will have ongoing losses in her urine, so you need to figure those in." ONGOING LOSSES, I wrote carefully. NEED TO ADD THEM IN.

My beeper went off. I pushed the button to stop it and looked at the extension on the display. I was being paged to Ten East, the adolescent ward where my team was based. As Paula worked on her senior admission note, I reached for a phone and punched in the number. The charge nurse, the head nurse for the shift, wanted me to know that there was a problem with one of the patients—she was threatening to leave.

"Which one?" I asked. I picked up my clipboard and took off the "signouts" that the other interns had given me before they'd left for the night, lists of their patients with the information I needed to take care of them overnight.

"Indy Martin."

Indy Martin, Indy Martin. I flipped through the sheets of paper until I found her name. She was a sixteen-year-old girl admitted two days before with a high fever and abdominal pain, later diagnosed as pyelonephritis, an infection in her kidneys. She had responded well to intravenous antibiotics, and I had thought that the plan made on rounds that morning was to discharge her with instructions to take antibiotics for another week.

Clearly I was forgetting something. "Why can't she leave?" I asked.

The charge nurse sounded annoyed. "Because DSS has nowhere to put her. They have been calling foster homes all day, and nobody wants her."

Suddenly I remembered what Indy's intern had told us when Indy was admitted. Her parents had decided about a year before that they couldn't handle her anymore and had put her into the custody of the Department of Social Services. She had lived in several foster homes since then; she kept running away for days or weeks at a time. DSS had put her in a psychiatric hospital because they felt she was depressed. Besides, no foster home was willing to take her. She had become sick while she was there, and the hospital had sent her to Children's. They didn't want her back, either.

I put my hand over the receiver and asked Paula what I should do. She shrugged and said to tell the charge nurse that I would be up to the ward as soon as I finished the admission. This wasn't quite the advice I was looking for; I was hoping she would tell me what to do about Indy. Not wanting to appear unable to deal with the situation, I did what she said.

I wrote a few more things on my index card about treating diabetic ketoacidosis. INSULIN DRIP, I wrote. REGULAR INSULIN, .1 UNITS PER KILOGRAM PER HOUR. POTASSIUM REPLACEMENT. I stared at the card. As a medical student I'd had lots of cards like this one, filled with all sorts of medical information. I had carried them around with me in my white coat but hadn't really needed them to take care of patients. Whenever I was writing orders a resident was always with me, who knew exactly what to do. Now I was the resident, and the card held new significance. I put it into my pocket and went with Paula to see the patient.

The mother of the diabetic girl was sitting on a chair next to the stretcher where her daughter lay. She was a small Asian woman who seemed too young to have a teenage daughter. She wore a faded blue cotton jacket over a wrinkled, rather worn green print dress. Her skin was a delicate light brown, and her short hair was very black, without any gray. She looked tired and worried, but resigned. Andrea had done this before, she told us. Whenever she got upset about anything she stopped taking her insulin. This time was worse than usual; she just hadn't been paying as much attention to Andrea as she should have been, she guessed. She knew about the trouble with her boyfriend, but, well, they were always fighting, and this fight didn't seem any different from the others.

Andrea lay on the stretcher, half sleeping, half watching her mother talk. Her skin was lighter, but she had inherited her mother's small, attractive features. Her long shiny hair fell across the pillow. She was skinny; her collarbones stuck out over the top of the hospital gown, and her elbows, hips, and knees were clearly visible under the sheet. I tried to ask her a few questions, but I couldn't make out her answers; she turned away from me and closed her eyes.

"I've never seen her like this," said her mother.

Paula and I asked the mother more questions about Andrea's medical history and what had happened, and then we examined her. We worked together, trying not to get in each other's way; we checked her from head to toe, looking, listening, and feeling. All we found were signs of dehydration: a fast heart rate, dry mouth, and skin that felt a little loose.

We finished, went back to the charting area, sat amid the books, papers, and phones, and wrote the admission orders for the medications, fluids, monitors, and tests that we wanted her to have. As we finished, Paula looked at her watch. She had stayed late to do the admission with me so that the senior who was covering for the night could take care of a sick child on the other ward team, but now she clearly wanted to go home. "Any questions?" she asked.

I wanted her to go over everything again with me, all the fluid management, all the instructions about potassium and insulin and dextrose. Even though I had it all written down, I felt scared and unsure and certain that somehow I wasn't going to be able to get it right.

"No," I said. "I'm all set."

On the way back to Ten East I stopped at the soda machine and bought a diet Coke. I went into the call room, after looking around to be sure nobody had seen me, and shut the door. It was a tiny, cramped room that barely held a bunk bed, a bedside table with a phone and a lamp on top, and a sink. It felt like a stuffy closet, but at least I was alone. I sat on the bottom bunk and drank the can of soda.

This was the night I had been looking forward to and fearing since I started medical school—and now it had arrived: my first night on call. I was the doctor for the team tonight.

I wasn't really alone. The senior on call was only a page away. But I couldn't page her every time I was paged or asked a question, and if it was a real emergency, I would have to make some decisions before I could get her help.

Had I learned enough in medical school? I didn't feel as though I had, especially not this night. I had learned about diabetes when we studied endocrinology in the second year of medical school, and I understood the physiology and bio-chemistry of diabetic ketoacidosis. Still, I had never taken care of a patient who had it. That was the random element of medical education during the clinical years: despite teaching conferences, we learned the most from the patients we took care of, and even though they tried to assign us patients to cover all the conditions we needed to learn about, it didn't always work out perfectly. As for Indy . . . I had had a rotation in psychiatry during my third year, but they hadn't taught us what to do with patients like Indy.

I had just completed four long years of medical school, yet suddenly I felt unprepared. There was an M.D. after my name, but I felt like a fraud. Despite all the studying and the clerkships, it seemed like I still had much to learn about medicine; I didn't feel ready for the responsibility of actually being a doctor.

My beeper went off; Ten East again. I threw the empty soda can into the trash, left the call room, and walked down the hall to the ward. As I approached I could hear someone yelling, and I saw two security guards and several nurses outside one of the rooms, looking in.

"There's going to be blood everywhere!" said the voice from inside the room. "Blood everywhere, I'm tellin ya!"

I worked my way through the little crowd behind the security guards and looked into the room. Indy was pacing back and forth. Her battered suitcase was on her bed, and she was dressed to go. She wore a black leather jacket with a skull and a bloody dagger painted on the back, tight blue jeans, and what looked like work boots spray-painted black. The roots of her long, rough hair were dark brown, almost black, but the rest of it was white blond.

The charge nurse, Rita, tapped me on the shoulder. She was short, with curly, shoulder-length hair and big glasses.

"I had to call Security," she told me. "She started walking down the hall with her suitcase, and when Helen and I tried to stop her she started hitting us."

"Are you okay?"

"Yeah, we're fine. It was more show than anything else.

But I was worried that the next time it wouldn't be, so I called these guys."

I watched Indy pacing. She was saying things under her breath; the few words I could make out were obscenities.

"Do we call DSS again?" I asked.

"Already did," said Rita. "They said there's nothing more they can do tonight. They'll start making calls again in the morning."

"Should I try talking to her?" I asked. I had no idea what I should say to her—but I was the doctor on call, so I figured I should do something.

"Be my guest. But be careful."

I put my clipboard on the desk and walked past the security guards into the room, or at least into the entrance. Indy stopped pacing and stood facing me, her hands on her hips. She was big for sixteen; she was a little overweight, but she was also just big—tall, with broad shoulders, heavy arms. She wore dark eye shadow and purple lipstick, and her hair hung across her face. She glared at me, and I was glad that the security guards were there. I took a step forward.

"Who are you?"

"I'm the doctor. My name is Claire McCarthy."

"You're not my doctor."

"I'm one of the doctors on the team. I'm the one who's here for the night."

"You gonna tell me why I can't leave?"

"Because there is nowhere for you to go."

"I got lotsa places to go. Don't give me that shit." She threw an empty soda can against the wall, hard. One of the security guards came into the room. I motioned to him to go back out.

"You think those guys scare me? I could hurt them bad."

I didn't say anything. I didn't know what to say.

"So why can't I leave?"

"You have to go home with someone, like to a foster home."

"I don't wanna go to no foster home. They are all shit-holes. I just wanna leave. I'm okay to leave, right? That's what my doctor told me."

"You're okay to leave medically, but there has to be some-place for you to go."

"Look, I told you. I got places to go. I got friends." Her voice was rising. I took a step back. I had no idea what I was doing, no plan for the situation at all. Indy kicked the wall, methodically and hard. I sat down on the chair by the door. There was a long silence.

"Look, Indy, I'm stuck," I said finally. "I understand why you want to leave. I would, too, if I were you. But I can't just let you out on the streets of Boston. I know you say you have friends who would look after you, and you probably do. But I can't let you go."

"I'd be fine." The kicking continued.

"I can't do it, Indy. I wish I could, but I can't."

"Yeah, right."

"No, really. Besides the fact that I'm not allowed to let you leave without consent from DSS, there's the fact that if I let you out on the streets around here, especially at night, you could be attacked. I wish I could change things, but I can't."

Indy stopped kicking and looked at me. Her arms were folded in front of her chest, and she looked right into my eyes with one of the most cynical, angry, and sad expressions I'd ever seen.

"You don't wish you could change anything," she said.

She's only sixteen years old, I thought. Sixteen years old, and she's looking at me like this. I felt a wave of sadness and tenderness for her.

"Yes, I do," I said. She looked at me for a few seconds more, then turned back to the wall.

"It's just one night," I said. I could sense Indy weighing her options.

"DSS gonna let me out in the morning?"

"I'm sure they will." I prayed I was telling the truth.

"I gotta think about it."

"Okay, you think about it." I got up.

"Hey."

"Yes?"

"Can I have a cigarette?"

"Sorry, there's no smoking in the hospital."

"There's no fuckin' place in this entire hospital where I can have a cigarette? There's no way I'm stayin'."

I looked at her and tried not to smile. "Okay, there's a smoking room. I'll tell the guards to take you there." It seemed like a reasonable bargain.

"What, I have to go with those jerks?"

"Yep, sorry."

"Oh, well," she said, and sighed. "The short one is kinda cute."

I went out and told the security guards to take her to the smoking room. I looked at the shorter guard. He was very dark, with a muscular build and a curly mustache. Not my type, I thought, but she was right. He looked at me questioningly; I smiled and walked away.

I went to check on Andrea. She had been brought up from the emergency room and was in one of the two-bed rooms close to the nurses' station, in the bed nearer the door. The cardiac monitor showed that her heart was still beating faster than normal, a sign that she was still dehydrated. Fluids and insulin ran through an infusion pump into the IV catheter in her left arm. Her eyes were closed, and she was still. I couldn't tell if she was sleeping.

Helen, one of the Ten East nurses, came up and stood next to me as I looked at Andrea.

"She's pretty sick, huh? Why didn't she go to the unit?"

Great, I thought. My first patient with diabetic ketoacidosis, and she is so sick with it that she should have gone to the intensive care unit.

"I don't know." It hadn't even occurred to me. I didn't know how those decisions were made. They told me to admit her, and I did.

"I was about to page you. Here are her last numbers."

She showed me a flow sheet with vital signs, medications, and lab values from blood and urine. The most recent lab values showed that she was still far from being in balance. Despite the therapy she had received so far, her blood sugar was still high and the chemicals in her blood were still out of balance.

I wasn't sure what Helen wanted me to say. We'd only just admitted her. Wasn't she allowed to stay sick for a while?

"I guess we'll just have to keep on with what we're doing," I said.

Helen frowned. "Did you see her potassium?"

So that's what she wanted. I looked at the lab values on the flow sheet again. Her potassium level was a little low. It wasn't dangerously low, which was why my eyes had passed over it when I looked at the flow sheet, but Helen was right to point it out. It was only going to get lower as she passed more out through her urine.

"Would you like me to add some to her IV fluid?" asked Helen.

Sounded like a good idea. "Sure."

"How much?"

I tried to think. How much would she need? I tried to do calculations in my head, taking into account her current level, her total body water, the amount of fluid she was getting, her urinary losses . . . Helen looked impatient, so I guessed.

"Ten milliequivalents per five hundred cc's?"

Helen gave me a look that I was starting to recognize as a "these new interns, they don't know anything" look. Hers wasn't unpleasant, though, just a little exasperated.

"Don't you think we should give a little more?"

Obviously she knew how much to give. I was relieved.

"What do you think we should do?" I asked.

"How about twenty per five hundred?"

"Fine," I said, and wrote the order on the order sheet.

I went back down the hall to the call room to change into the scrub shirt and pants that I had found on the linen cart. I folded my clothes and put them on the top bunk. My pens and "code card" with the doses of all the drugs it might be necessary to use in an emergency went into the front pocket of the scrub top. I tied the drawstring pants tightly, put my beeper on the waistband, and looked at myself in the mirror. I didn't look any different from when I'd worn scrubs as a medical student. I started out the door but then stopped; I sat on the bed, pulled out my code card, and tried to memorize at least a few of the medicine doses, just in case. The words and numbers swam in my head; it was useless. I went back to the ward to work on progress and admission notes.

The senior on call for the night, Cheryl, stopped by to see how things were going. Forcing a smile, I said that everything was fine. I asked if Andrea was particularly sick for someone with diabetic ketoacidosis, sick enough to go to the intensive care unit.

"Actually," said Cheryl, "yes. She's borderline. But they are so tight on beds in the unit that they asked if there was any way she could go to the floor instead. Don't worry, though—you're doing fine with her. Just page me if you have any questions." She turned and walked out toward the elevators. As I watched her, I wondered if I would ever be able to walk the way she did, with such confidence.

A couple of the nurses asked me some questions about a few of the patients. They were only little questions, but I could answer them, and that made me feel good. As I finished with them, Helen motioned to me to come over to Andrea's room.

"Just wanted to show you the latest glucose."

I looked at where she was pointing on the flow sheet. Andrea's blood sugar, or glucose, was now two hundred and ten. That was down quite a bit.

"Great!" I said.

"Do you want to make any changes in her fluids?"

I reached into my scrub shirt pocket for my index card, only to find that I had left it in the call room. Okay. I was supposed to put dextrose back into the IV fluid when her blood sugar was less than . . . what? Was it two hundred? Two hundred and fifty?

Helen rescued me. "Usually we go to five percent dextrose when the glucose is less than three hundred."

"Thanks," I said, and wrote the order. I didn't feel particularly good anymore. I got my index card from the call room and went back to writing my notes.

I finished at around one in the morning and decided to walk around the ward to see if anything was happening before I went to bed. I heard muffled rock music coming from the activity room down the hall. The shorter security guard was standing outside the door.

I went over to him. "How are things?"

"She seems to be quieting down. We decided one of us was enough."

"And you were the lucky one?"

"Well, she seemed to get along with me a little better, so

we thought it would be better for me to stay. You know, she might listen to me more than him."

I smiled. "I bet she would." I looked into the room; the lights were off. "What is she doing in there?"

"Just listening to her tape. I keep checking on her, don't worry. She said she wanted the lights out."

"I'm going to go in, okay?"

He nodded. "I'll be watching. Just yell if you need me."

As I opened the door slowly and went in, the music was almost deafening. It was hard rock, heavy metal stuff. It took a few seconds for my eyes to adjust to the darkness. Indy was sitting on the wide windowsill, looking out. It was a huge window that looked out over Boston; the Prudential building, the Hancock building and all the others were silhouetted against the darkness sprinkled with light.

"Indy?" She didn't answer. "Indy?"

I went over to the stereo and turned down the volume. She turned around and jumped off the windowsill.

"It's just me," I said.

She sat back down and looked out the window again. I went over and sat on the windowsill a few feet down from her.

"What are you looking at?"

She motioned down, toward the front of the hospital. "I'm waitin' for someone."

"Who?"

"I got this friend, and he knows I'm here so he's gonna come get me out."

"Oh?"

"Yeah. I seen his car driving by a coupla times. He's just waitin' for a good time, then he'll be here."

I looked down. The semicircular area in front of the hospital was empty except for three darkened parked cars. Out on Longwood Avenue a few cars passed by, mostly taxicabs.

"He's got a limo," said Indy. "He's in the Mafia."

"How do you know him?"

She shrugged. "I just do, that's all. He's gonna come get me, you'll see. They won't be able to stop him down there."

We both looked out the window for a while. I didn't see any limousines.

She got up, went over to the stereo, and turned the volume back up. The harsh guitar and drums filled the room. She stood by the stereo and danced with her back to me, her broad hips swaying back and forth. There was something about the way she danced that made me wonder how she supported herself when she ran away.

I got off the windowsill and went to the door. "Good night," I said, but she didn't hear me.

Back in the call room I shut the door behind me and turned off the light. I put my stethoscope and beeper on the bedside table and crawled under the blanket with my sneakers on. I wanted to be ready if anything happened.

I dreamed that more nurses than I could count were showing me flow sheets filled with numbers. "Look at this!" they were saying. "No, look at this!" "No, this!" I tried to run away, but the two security guards who had been watching Indy stopped me and dragged me back.

I awoke with a start and sat up, almost hitting my head on the top bunk. I looked at my watch: five minutes after seven. I splashed water on my face, picked up my beeper and stethoscope, and walked quickly to the ward. Had nothing really happened for the rest of the night?

The nurses' station was bustling; it was change of shift. I went by Andrea's room and looked at her flow sheet. The numbers looked terrific, almost back to normal. She was back in balance. I went into the room. She was sitting up in bed, watching television.

"How are you feeling?"

"Much better, thanks." She smiled. "I'm sorry I was so much trouble." It was the same tiny voice as the night before, but it was stronger now. Everything about her seemed stronger, and her eyes were brighter. They were beautiful eyes, chocolate brown with long eyelashes. She had combed her hair, and it lay delicately against her shoulders.

"You weren't. I'm glad you're feeling better."

I suddenly thought of those dehydrated meals you take when you go camping. You add water, and the drab dry stuff becomes Stroganoff or something. I looked at her and thought, We added water, and we got this lovely girl. I laughed.

"What's funny?"

"Oh, nothing. Can I get you anything?"

"How about breakfast?"

"We'll see. We need to be sure your body is ready for you to eat. Okay?"

Andrea nodded and went back to watching television.

She really is better, I thought. She was very sick, sick enough that she could have died, and now she's better. I couldn't really take credit for it, since I'd simply done what Paula and Helen had told me to do, but I'd helped. I'd helped, and I'd learned how to take care of someone with diabetic ketoacidosis. Although I'd known that's how the apprenticeship of residency worked, experiencing it made me feel relieved. Maybe I'd be okay after all.

There was a different security guard sitting on a chair outside Indy's room. I nodded to him and peeked inside. Indy was curled up on her side, fast asleep, with her blanket pulled up under her chin. She looked sweet and childlike. Medical school couldn't prepare me for everything anyway, I thought as I looked at her. There are some things I'm going to have to figure out as I go along.

WELL CHILD
CARE

*T*hey give us an exam room with a place outside the door where we can put the nameplate they made for us, supply us with crib sheets on what we are supposed to ask and do at well child care visits, show us our list of patients, and we become pediatricians.

We are completely unprepared as interns to do this. Although we all studied pediatrics during medical school, very few of us did much outpatient work. After spending four years learning how to take care of the sick, especially the hospitalized sick, in this part of residency we are supposed to know how to take care of the well. It sounds as though it should be easy, but it's not.

"*I* want a young doctor, someone who's up on stuff, you know?" Donna said to me while I was taking care of her two-month-old daughter, Jessica, during her admission for a skin infection. "The pediatrician we've been going to, well, he's kind of an old fart."

I tried not to smile, if only out of professional courtesy.

"Do you have patients? I mean, do you only work on this floor or do you give shots and stuff, too?"

A little surprised, I told her that no, I didn't always work on the inpatient wards, that one afternoon a week I saw patients in clinic.

She looked at me brightly. "Are you taking new patients?"

"Sure," I said, and we arranged appointments for Jessica and her older child.

*T*hey arrived on time, my only patients of the afternoon, toting all their paraphernalia: a stroller, a huge baby bag, and a baby carrier. Donna came without her husband—he's working, she explained—and I watched with amazement as she managed to carry everything and maneuver down the hallway. I offered to help.

"No, that's okay," she said with a smile. "I'm fine."

She walked ahead of me into the room and put the baby carrier holding Jessica, now almost three months, on the chair. She put the baby bag on the floor and let Bobby, eighteen months, out of the stroller. Immediately he ran under the examination table and sat down.

"Fine," said Donna. She pulled out two toy trucks from the bag. "Play with these." She rolled them under the exam table. Bobby picked them up and started to bang them together and on the floor, saying "vroom, vroom" over and over.

Above the din, Donna proceeded to tell me that she was worried about Jessica because she was always throwing up.

"It's like all the time," she told me. "Every time I feed her, she pukes. Gets all over the place. It's usually a lot, and it's *all* the time. I thought maybe it was 'cause she didn't like the iron in the formula, so I tried the low-iron kind, but it didn't make any difference."

I asked all the usual medical questions. Jessica never had a fever, she didn't have diarrhea or constipation, she didn't cry a lot, she never threw up bile, she wasn't coughing, she didn't have any rashes—there didn't seem to be anything else wrong with her. I looked at her weight, written down by the assistant who had weighed her. She had gained weight since her discharge from the hospital. She hadn't gained much—I would have liked to see her weigh a little more— but she had gained.

"Bobby used to puke, but that's 'cause I was feeding him too much. Once I cut down, he was fine."

I hadn't thought of overfeeding as a possible cause; it certainly made sense. "How much do you feed Jessica?"

"Oh, not too much. I wouldn't do that again. She only takes about four or five ounces."

Four or five ounces. Was that too much? Was that enough? I was embarrassed not to know. It seemed okay, and she seemed sure of herself, so I let it pass.

I did the usual physical exam on Jessica, and she appeared to be completely healthy. She even smiled at me, showing off her gums and drool.

I didn't know what to say about the vomiting. I had heard that some babies tend to spit up. I said this to Donna.

"This isn't just the usual baby spit-up," she said. "This is more."

Not knowing exactly how much spit-up could be classified as usual, I told her that Jessica seemed to be healthy.

"My friend's baby did the same thing as Jessica, the throwing up, I mean," said Donna. "She mixed some rice cereal in with his formula—not a lot, just a little to make it heavier in his stomach. Worked real well. Could I try that?"

I thought about it. I hadn't heard of it before, but it didn't seem like a dangerous thing to do. It didn't involve spoon feeding, for which Jessica was clearly too young, and although I had been taught that babies weren't supposed to start solids until four months, rice cereal is fairly gentle on the intestines. Maybe if Donna did this, more formula *would* stay in her stomach and she would gain more weight.

"Sure," I said. "Why not?"

At the next appointment Jessica's weight gain was perfect. I asked about the vomiting.

"Oh, that went away as soon as I started adding the rice cereal," she said. "Now it's just usual baby spit-up."

*D*onna called me often. Almost a third of the times my beeper went off when I was out of the hospital, it was she. Every once in a while, it was what I classified as a worthwhile call, like for a high fever or a bad fall. Most of the time, though, the calls seemed to be about issues I found incredibly minor.

I remember one call that I had to get out of the shower to answer.

"Jessica's got a fever," she told me. "It's just a little fever and I know it's from her cold 'cause she's got a really runny nose and a little cough. It's not a bad cold, though."

"Yes?" I said, dripping on the living room floor.

"Can I give her Tylenol?"

"What?"

"Can I give her Tylenol? I mean, I know you told me to give it to her if she got a fever with her shots, but can I give it to her for this fever, too? She's not too young, is she?"

If I said she could get it for fever, why did she need to call me? I decided not to ask.

"Sure, you can give her Tylenol. Let me know if the fever

doesn't go away or if she gets sicker. Bye." I was making a puddle on the wood floor.

"Wait!" she said.

"Yes?"

"Do I give her the same amount you told me to?"

"Yes."

"Okay. Thanks!" she said, and hung up.

As I climbed back into the shower, I felt annoyed. It seemed to me perfectly self-explanatory that Tylenol would help bring a fever down no matter what its cause. But then again, I thought as I reached for the shampoo, "usual baby spit-up" was self-explanatory to her, and I had yet to figure out what that was.

She brought Bobby in a few weeks after his second birthday because she was sure he had an ear infection.

"Does he have a fever?"

"No."

"Has he been pulling at his ear?"

"No."

"Then why do you think he has an ear infection?"

" 'Cause I can tell."

Bobby sat solemnly on the exam table, staring at me.

I looked in his ears. Sure enough, his left ear was infected. I helped him off the table and wrote a prescription for an antibiotic, which I handed to Donna.

"I've been meaning to ask you," said Donna.

"Yes?"

"We've been having problems with Jessica lately. She used to sleep through the night, but now she wakes up crying in the middle of the night. It's been happening every night, and it's driving me and my husband crazy."

"Is she acting sick?"

"No, she's not sick or anything, and there's nothing different at home, either. It's just at night. We can get her to go back to sleep, but only if we bring her into bed with us, and I don't want to keep doing that."

I hadn't learned anything about this; it hadn't come up in medical school or residency. I didn't know what to say. While I was trying to come up with a way to hide my ignorance, Donna said, "I think I know why she might be doing it."

"Why?"

"Well, she's nine months old now, and she's starting to want us when we're not there, you know what I mean? Before it was like she forgot about us when she couldn't see us—as long as she had something to do or someone to play with, she didn't care if we left. Now she does care. I think she misses us at night."

This sounded familiar. It sounded like something I had read about called "object permanence," the realization that something or someone exists even when out of sight. If I remembered right, nine months was in the age range for this developmental milestone.

"So maybe she just needs to know that you are there."

"Yeah, she does stop crying when one of us goes in the room, but as soon as we leave she starts again. That's why we end up bringing her into our bed."

"If you keep doing that, it will become a habit for her, and she won't be able to go back to sleep in her own bed," I said. I was drawing on common sense rather than pediatric knowledge, but I tried to say it with authority.

"But I can't stand it when she cries!"

We talked some more and worked out a plan. Either she or her husband would go in and comfort her, then leave. They would let her cry for a little while and then go back in and comfort her again, trying to wait a little longer each time before going back in. That way she would know that her parents were there and that they would respond to her crying, but she would learn to fall back to sleep in her crib rather than their bed. It was a negotiated plan and mostly Donna's idea.

"It's worth a try," said Donna.

I called her the following week to see how things were going.

"The first couple of nights were hell," she said. "I was starting to think there was no way it could work. But it's much better now. We've had two nights where she's slept all night, and the other nights we can usually get her to stop and go back to sleep just by patting her and shushing her."

A couple of months later in our teaching session before clinic, we learned about the ideas of Dr. Ferber, a Children's staff pediatrician and expert on pediatric sleep problems. One of the examples given was that of a nine-month-old who had previously slept through the night but suddenly was waking up and crying—exactly Jessica's story. And the plan of treatment that Dr. Ferber suggested was almost exactly the plan Donna had come up with.

She taught me so much. There are practical realities of taking care of children that are not part of the curriculum in medical school. What do you do if a child refuses to take medicines? For that matter, which medicines taste okay and which taste horrible? How much do babies eat? How do you mix formula? What do you use for a standard diaper rash? How do you toilet train a child? How do you get them to switch from the bottle to the cup? The list went on and on.

I marveled at how much Donna knew, and knew easily,

naturally. Once I asked her how she had learned something, I can't remember what it was now, and she laughed.

"Oh, I don't know," she said. "Did my mother tell me that one? No, I think it was one of my friends. We all sit around and talk about our kids, you know, and about what stuff works and all that."

It dawned on me that most young mothers are part of a community of mothers: their own mothers, their sisters, their friends with children. It is a community that nurtures and teaches, a community that most of us in our pediatric residency had little or no access to. Most of us had postponed parenthood because of the demands of becoming physicians, many of us had moved away from our families at some point in our education, and although there were exceptions, most of our friends were professionals who had also postponed parenthood.

I listened carefully to the stories Donna told about situations at home and the way she dealt with them. I paid attention to the things she pulled out of the diaper bag. I watched closely when she changed a diaper or gave Jessica her bottle. There was so much to learn.

At the beginning of my senior year, Donna had a third child, a boy named Billy, and she and her husband moved to a community farther away from Boston. She talked with me about using a pediatrician closer to home for shots and minor things, since it was a long drive from their new home to Children's and it would be difficult with three small children.

"If they are really sick, though, I want to come here," she said.

I said that it wasn't fair to the local pediatrician, and that anyway she should be going to someone she trusted with everything, not just shots. She said she'd think about it. What ended up happening was that after she started going to the new pediatrician she would call me, to "okay" things, to run them by me. I tried to discourage it, but Donna was very persistent, and at any rate it didn't last very long.

"Billy is vomiting," she called me to tell me. "Every time I feed him, he vomits."

"Is it the usual baby spit-up?" I asked.

"No, no, it's more. I think it's the formula. It's not the iron 'cause I tried the low-iron kind. I think he needs a different brand."

"Is he sick? Does he have fevers or diarrhea?"

"No, he's fine. And I'm not feeding him too much. He's just vomiting."

"Have you talked with your new pediatrician about this?"

"No, not yet. I know, I should. But I think it's the formula—I want to change. Which one should I change to?"

"Have you thought about mixing some rice cereal in with the formula?"

"No. I don't think it's the same as it was with Jessica. I think he doesn't like the formula."

I told her I doubted she needed to change the formula. She seemed annoyed, and the conversation ended abruptly.

A few weeks later she called to run something else by me. At the end of the conversation she said, "Oh, by the way, Billy's not vomiting anymore."

"Really? What was it that helped?"

"Well, I changed the formula a couple of times, but he still vomited, so I tried mixing in some rice cereal and that helped a lot."

"I'm glad he stopped."

"Yeah, my mother told me I should have listened to you in the first place. After all, you are a doctor."

ARTHUR

Arthur was a premature baby, born at twenty-three weeks, who made the mistake of crying in the delivery room.

His mother had gone into labor, and the obstetricians were unable to stop it. Nobody expected the baby to live. The parents were prepared for what they were thinking of as a miscarriage, and the pediatric resident was called to the delivery room out of formality more than anything else. She was expected to pronounce the baby dead or at least unable to be resuscitated.

But Arthur came out crying. And given that he had made that statement—expressed a desire to try living—the pediatric resident felt that she had no choice but to insert a breathing tube and bring him to the neonatal intensive care unit. I don't blame her, really; it is very hard to let a crying baby die. It may be the right thing to do, but it is very hard.

From the very beginning, it was a struggle to keep him alive. He actually had amazing lungs for a premature child —or rather a fetus—but nothing else worked very well. He was simply not ready to be born. His skin peeled and tore, his blood pressure was too low, he had problems maintaining the normal chemicals in his blood, and he constantly needed transfusions.

But he held on. When he was born his eyes were fused shut, but one day they opened, and he became a little person. Most of the time he was too sick to have much of a personality, but when he was more stable, he did. He was active and feisty and loved to suck on his very tiny pacifier.

His parents, Diane and Joe, were in their forties. Diane was a small, thin Asian woman who wore her hair pulled tightly back from her elegant face. She had a degree in molecular biology and worked in a lab at a local university where Joe was an English professor. She held herself rigidly, and whenever I told her bad news about Arthur, she stiffened, visibly steeled herself.

Joe was different. Tall and gangly, with a graying beard, he had a loud laugh and an easy manner. He was open and unprotected; he could accept bad news, but he could not steel himself. One day when they were visiting, they told me how neither of them had expected to marry, let alone have a child. They had thought themselves loners, too caught up in their work. But then they met and fell in love, and suddenly they wanted very much to have a child.

When Arthur was just under three weeks old his intestine perforated, a common problem in babies that premature, and he went to the operating room for repair. At that point he had dropped from his birth weight of six hundred and eighty grams to about five hundred grams, a little more than a pound. He was stable for a little while after the operation, but soon it became clear that he might be too tiny to save. He was too tiny to get IVs into, and his body couldn't tolerate any more than 5 percent dextrose, which was entirely inadequate nutrition to make him grow. He was experiencing one complication after another.

I guess we had an opportunity to stop when his intestine perforated, but we didn't use it. I suppose it was because he had done relatively well until then, or at least relatively well for his extreme prematurity. And also, as is so often the case in neonatology or medicine in general, we were focused on fixing the immediate problem as opposed to considering the ramifications of fixing it.

We had a family meeting. I was there, as Arthur's primary intern, along with the primary nurse and one of the neonatologists. We talked about how sick Arthur was and how we didn't know what would happen with him or whether we could make him better. We talked about our immediate goals of clearing the infection that had developed and getting him to gain weight, and we talked about the possible need to redirect our care toward comfort measures if we were unsuccessful and not try to make him better anymore.

Diane talked, too. "I hate myself for saying this," she said, "but I'm starting to resent my own son. It's just been so hard, with him being so sick, and not knowing."

She looked down at her hands folded on the conference table in front of her. "And you know, I don't know if I could really deal with it and take care of him if he ended up handicapped or brain damaged as you guys say he might."

She looked up at us. "It's not that I don't love him. I do love him, really. It's just that I know what my limits are. And I still have things I want to do with my life."

Joe seemed very uncomfortable. He looked at Diane with a strange mixture of anger, frustration, and understanding. He shrugged. "I guess I don't quite agree with my wife," he said. "Arthur is my son, and I want to keep him in whatever condition he ends up in." He paused for a moment and frowned. "Unless he was going to be some kind of vegetable, then it wouldn't be worth it. If he didn't have a personality—if you could tell me or I could see that he had lost his personality—then I think I'd want to stop."

We set a week from that day as a time to talk again, to reevaluate, but Arthur didn't give us that long. I was on call the night he got very sick. It came on insidiously but with certainty; he was overwhelmingly infected despite antibiotics, and his kidneys were failing. Arthur was not just giving us an opportunity, he was making our decision for us.

What is it that frightens us so about death? Why can't there be some beauty in allowing it, in letting it happen and be peaceful? Why do we as physicians have so much trouble giving in? We should have let Arthur die long before he did.

At about six in the morning I called Diane and Joe and asked them to come to the hospital. They sat with the senior neonatologist and me in the conference room with its pictures of mothers and babies on the walls. I told them what had happened and that the only things we could do were extraordinary measures and temporizing at best.

"It's up to you," the senior neonatologist said to them, "but we would favor withdrawing support."

Diane and Joe held hands in the grim quiet.

"When you called," Joe said, "we knew what it was about." He looked at Diane, who looked back at him and squeezed his hand.

"We talked about it on the way over," he continued quietly, "and we decided that Arthur has been through enough already." His voice broke on the last word, and his eyes filled with tears. Diane looked relieved but very, very sad.

They each held him for a few minutes while he was still on the ventilator that breathed for him. We weren't sure how long he would live after we removed the breathing tube.

Then they went to the family room to wait, and Jenny, the primary nurse, and I were left with the task of disconnecting and untaping. Whereas before Arthur had been markedly lethargic, he began to be more alert, to open his eyes and look around. Jenny began to cry and left the room. I think it was harder for her than it was for me. She had cared for him and been with him for many hours at a time, many days in a row. She knew him better than anyone in the intensive care unit.

The charge nurse helped me, and together we took out the IVs, disconnected the leads, and turned off the monitors. I gave him a nice large dose of morphine. It wasn't enough to stop him from breathing, but it was enough to take away any pain or agitation he might have been feeling. The last thing we did was take out his breathing tube. In the last moments of his life he was bundled up for the first time in the way babies are usually bundled up.

Jenny came back, and we took Arthur to his parents. We left them to hold him. It was the first time they had ever held him unhooked, the first—and last—time they were ever together as a family.

I came in fifteen minutes later. They were both crying.

"I think he's dead," Joe said.

I put on my stethoscope and listened to his chest; it was silent. I took off the stethoscope.

"His heart isn't beating anymore," I said. They were very quiet. I felt as though I should say something, but it was hard.

"He was a beautiful child," I said, "and I'm sure that he knew you loved him."

They were still very quiet. Joe held Diane as she held Arthur.

"Would you like to hold him some more," I asked, "or would you like me to take him?"

They looked at each other, and finally Diane said, "You can take him."

There was a bassinet in the room, but I couldn't bear to wheel him out in it, so I took him in my arms and left them. I brought him and the bassinet into the triage room across the hall and went over to the corner of the room. He was so light; it was as if I were carrying nothing at all. I stood there in the corner of the room, holding the little dead baby, and I didn't know what to do. I didn't want to leave him. I held him close to me and kissed him on the forehead and laid him carefully in the bassinet. I looked at the clock because the senior neonatologist had told me I would need to have a time of death. I had never pronounced anyone dead before.

It was soft, his death; it was like a slipping away. And he was held, as we all should be when we die.

He was simply not ready to be in this world. We had all known it in our hearts, but we had wanted to deny it, we had wanted to change it. We who are so powerful, we who manipulate physiology and life itself, are not very good at admitting that there are things we cannot change.

THE BABY'S

RASH

I couldn't understand anything anyone was
saying. Five adults were crammed into the little exam room
in the emergency room; a woman on a chair in the corner
was holding the baby. They were Brazilian, and nobody
seemed to speak anything but Portuguese. Sometimes I can
understand bits of Portuguese when the words sound like
Spanish words, but this time I couldn't make out anything.
Maybe it was because they were all talking at once.

The doctor who called from the local clinic that had sent
them in said that the baby, an eleven-month-old girl, had
been brought in by an aunt who had said, through an interpreter who worked at the clinic, that the baby had a rash.
She'd said she had no idea how long it had been there or
what might have caused it. The doctor had taken one look
at the rash and called Children's.

I asked if anyone spoke English. I got blank stares, and a
couple of people shook their heads. I asked if anyone spoke
Spanish. The response was the same. I decided to examine
the baby and then get an interpreter.

The woman in the corner holding the baby was heavy, with long thick wavy black hair tied back loosely with a rubber band. She wore an old blue denim jumper with a frayed T-shirt underneath, and sneakers. The baby was huddled in the woman's big arms, and she watched me closely and with suspicion. She had curly black hair that needed washing, and her red-and-white-checked dress was way too big for her.

"Mother?" I asked, pointing at the woman.

"No," she said with a frown. She paused and then said, "Ont." So she was the one who'd brought the baby to the clinic.

"Mother?" I asked, pointing at the other woman in the room, a very young woman in jeans, standing by the door.

"No," said the woman holding the baby. No explanation was offered this time. Everyone in the room was staring at me.

"Can I see her?" I asked slowly, motioning toward the stretcher.

The woman seemed to understand. She stood up and carried her over. The little girl looked at me with terrified eyes. It was kind of strange how scared she was.

The woman put her down on the stretcher, and she screamed.

"How about you sit with her?" I said, acting it out myself. The woman nodded and sat on the stretcher with the girl on her lap. She stopped crying, but her eyes were still scared.

I noticed something on the girl's wrist. Gently I took her hand and looked more closely. It looked like a bruise, and it went all around her wrist, about an inch or so wide. It looked old, and it looked like something, I couldn't think what. I looked at the other wrist—there was a similar bruise. There didn't seem to be anything else on her arms.

"Where is the rest of it?" I asked, pointing to the bruises and trying to look questioning.

The woman frowned and then seemed to understand. She pointed at the girl's legs and diaper area.

Carefully I lifted the dress, which fell below her knees, undid the diaper, and looked.

I was stunned.

The same bruises were present around her thighs. All of a sudden I knew what they were from—a rope. They were old rope burns. Someone had tied this baby down. And I could see what they had tied her down to do.

The area between her legs was one big bruise. Her labia were almost entirely purple, and when I looked at her vaginal opening, it was wider than it should have been for her age and scarred.

I went to touch her labia, to pull them apart some more to see if there was any other damage, and the little girl started to scream. It wasn't just a scream; I don't think I can convey how chilling it was. It was filled with fear and with desperation.

I had to leave the room because I was about to cry. I came back a few minutes later to finish the physical exam. I listened to her heart and lungs, felt her belly, checked her eyes, ears, and mouth. All of those were normal. I didn't speak as I worked; I couldn't speak. I stared at each and every one of the people there, all of whom looked at me blankly. I wondered if the person who had done this, who had raped this beautiful girl, was in the room. The very thought made me shake with anger and fear.

My shift finished before the interpreter came; I never got to hear what any of those people said.

*T*hat was the first case of abuse I saw and one of the most painful to see. I was an intern then, doing my first rotation through the emergency room, and I was unprepared for it. I should have realized that I would have to deal with child abuse as a pediatrician, but somehow I hadn't. There was more, much more, that I saw in the months I spent in the emergency room.

*T*he mother was young and nervous. She paced outside the exam room and almost jumped when I came over and introduced myself.

We went into the room together. A little boy was sitting on the stretcher, coloring in a coloring book. He was four years old.

"He told me something this morning," the mother said, taking a deep breath. The boy didn't look up. "He told me my husband touches his doolie—that's the word we use for penis."

"Wiping him after he goes to the bathroom?" I asked. "When he's getting a bath?"

The woman shook her head vigorously. "No," she said, "You don't understand. I take him to the bathroom and give him his bath. He says it's when my husband is reading him a story, and that he sometimes gets in bed with him. He says he touches it for a long time, and that it's supposed to be a secret."

The little boy still hadn't looked up. I knew he was listening, and I was uncomfortable. We should have talked somewhere else, I thought.

The woman looked at me, her eyes red and wet. "My daughter, she's seven, and you know, she's been acting really weird recently. I wonder if . . ."

I examined the little boy; his exam was normal. Not that I necessarily expected to find anything—simply touching the penis wouldn't leave anything to find.

I explained to the mother that she was going to have to talk to the social worker, and we were going to have to make some kind of plan for the children's safety while this was investigated further.

She looked at her watch. "I don't know," she said. "I have to get home before he does. He can't know I was here."

"Why?" I asked.

"He'd beat me up bad," she said. "He's done it before." She looked at the little boy, who had gone back to coloring. "I don't care so much about that, though. I'm just afraid he'd get angry and hurt him, too."

I just couldn't understand this, this hurting of children. It was unthinkable to me that someone would deliberately beat or molest a defenseless child. I'd read about it in the paper, but it had never seemed real, and I'd hoped it was rare. Within a few months of starting my residency, I found that it was very real and it wasn't rare.

And it was such a slippery thing sometimes, hard to prove or even describe. So often, it seemed, the perpetrators went unpunished; so often nothing changed.

*H*annah was her name. She had fine blond hair like corn silk that hung close around her head and hazel eyes with long lashes. She was thirteen years old but looked younger; she was tiny, thin, and delicate. She reminded me of the little dancers that go round and round inside a music box, the old-fashioned kind.

Her voice was tiny, too, but it was clear and sure as she

spoke. Her mother, Deirdre, sat on the stretcher next to her, her arms wrapped around her as though she were an infant again. Hannah must have looked like her father, for Deirdre was large and darker. They shared a delicateness, though, and a vulnerability.

Hannah was overwhelmed. I think she had never expected to end up in the emergency room when she told her mother about what had been happening. She'd been trying to get her alone for a long time, apparently, but her stepfather always seemed to be around.

With gentle coaxing, she told us that it had been going on for a long time. When it had started it hadn't seemed so bad. Her stepfather would get into bed with her when she was watching television in her room. At first he just put his arm around her or touched her leg, and she figured he was allowed to do that since he was her stepfather. Then he started touching her breasts and putting his hand between her legs. He didn't look at her; he'd just look at the television and touch her that way.

It scared her. She would sit there and not move. She didn't understand. She wanted to tell her mother, but she was afraid that she'd be angry. Once her mother came into the room, but he quickly took his hand away. She said it was nice that they were spending time together.

It kept happening, and then one night he took off her underwear and got on top of her, and it hurt, and then it was wet, and when she went into the bathroom afterward there was some blood.

Deirdre shuddered. She let go of Hannah for a second to wipe some tears and then held on to her even tighter.

After that Hannah stopped watching television and tried pretending that she was sick or asleep, hoping that he would leave her alone. It sort of worked, usually, but two other times he got on top of her and hurt her. The last time was last week.

She just didn't understand. He said it was his special way of showing how much he loved her. He said she was very beautiful. She thought maybe it was her fault, because she was beautiful or something.

"I just can't believe this," said Deirdre. "My husband, he's been so good to us, to both me and Hannah. He's a gentle man. He's given us so many nice things. He has provided for us in every way. My ex-husband was a real jerk. But Ed, he's so different. He's been a wonderful husband—and father."

With Deirdre close by, I examined Hannah. There weren't any cuts or bruises or other signs of trauma, not that her story suggested there should be. When I did her pelvic exam I used the kit we used for collecting evidence in cases of rape, although I knew that the yield would be low. It had been a week since the last episode, so I didn't think there would be any sperm or hairs or other evidence, but it was worth a try. I did cultures for gonorrhea and chlamydia, although there was no vaginal discharge to suggest infection. Her hymen was no longer intact, but otherwise her exam was normal. Without excessive use of force, though, it would be normal.

I asked Hannah if she ever used tampons. She said yes, a couple of times. Oh, well, I thought. That could be used by a defense lawyer to explain why her hymen wasn't intact.

All we had to go on was her word.

I sent them to the social worker, who took a more thorough history of the situation at home. She set up an appointment with the sexual abuse team for Hannah and convinced Deirdre that she and Hannah shouldn't go home, that they should stay with a friend for a while.

About two weeks later, Deirdre paged me. "I just wanted to ask you . . ." she said.

"Yes?"

"It's just that I talked with Ed, and he says that he never touched Hannah like that. He was really upset that I could even think it was true."

I didn't say anything.

"And you know, it got me wondering . . ." Her voice trailed off for a few seconds, then she continued with a little more resolve. "Maybe she's jealous of my relationship with Ed, maybe she misses her father, so she made up the story to get back at Ed."

"You think she made that up?" I was incredulous.

"You said yourself there wasn't any evidence." She paused. "It's just that Ed has been so good to us. He takes care of everything. I—I don't know if I could make it without him. And he says it's not true. You should have seen him. He almost cried."

"Kids don't make that kind of stuff up," I said.

"Hannah's really smart. And you know all the stuff that's on TV these days. Maybe she got the idea from some TV show."

I closed my eyes, and I could see Hannah huddled next to her mother on the stretcher, pushing her thin blond hair out of her face, telling her story in her clear, soft voice.

"I'm sorry," I said, "but I believe her. I believe every word she said. And I think you'd be making a horrible mistake if you don't believe her, too." I was so angry, I could barely get the words out.

There was a long silence before Deirdre spoke.

"Yeah, well, thanks," she said, and hung up.

There were just so many. There were the little babies who had been shaken so hard that their brains were damaged. There were children who had been beaten, or smothered, or badly hurt, some of whom died. There were the children with the burns or broken bones for which there were no good explanations.

Sometimes we were given explanations. He fell, they'd say; he's clumsy. She likes to play with the water in the shower, and she must have turned the hot water on herself. He was playing with the kids down the street—one of them must have hit him and that's how he broke his arm. And they would stick to the story, even though we couldn't imagine how he could have fallen to cause that bruise and they couldn't explain how the water from the shower could have fallen on that one place on her back and nowhere else and that particular kind of fracture in the arm is only seen in child abuse.

Sometimes they just looked at us blankly and said they had no idea how it happened. One mother of a shaken baby said absolutely nothing had happened; she'd brought the baby to the hospital simply because she was crying more than usual. A CAT scan of the baby's head showed severe damage; the baby had been shaken very hard.

It happens, I was told. People get stressed out or strung out or angry for whatever reason, and they lash out. It was unthinkable, so I tried not to think about it. It was easier to think about the medical issues only—dressing the burns, stopping the seizures caused by the brain damage, doing the cultures for gonorrhea on a three-year-old girl who had been raped—and to let the social workers and the Department of Social Services and the police think about the rest.

I didn't really stop thinking about it, of course; I thought about it all the time. Every time a parent brought a child in who'd had any kind of injury, I found myself asking all sorts of questions. I made them go over the story again and again, looking for incongruities or changes. I asked questions about who was in the house at the time. I asked all sorts of questions, questions I would have thought too personal to be appropriate before I started seeing abused children. I started watching the way parents told the story, watching the expressions on their faces. I watched the way they acted toward their children and the way their children acted toward them.

It wasn't just with the children who were there with injuries. I started watching all the parents and children, no matter what they were in the hospital for. I asked for explanations for every bruise or scar I found. I did careful genital examinations. I stopped trusting anyone.

And when I started looking so closely, I started seeing things that I didn't know quite what to make of or do about. Like children who looked as though nobody had washed them or changed their clothes in days, yet who were healthy and acted warmly toward their mothers. Or a mother who spoke very sharply to a child and spanked him—then picked him up and hugged him. Or a baby left entirely alone in a waiting room while a parent went to make a phone call. I'd ask questions of all of these parents, come up with nothing clearly abusive or neglectful that could be reported, and I'd wonder what I was missing.

Whenever we thought a child had been abused or neglected, we called the Department of Social Services, who investigated and took whatever action they deemed appropriate. But it often seemed that little could be done for abused or neglected children. Even if the abuse could be proved, there just didn't seem to be enough resources, staff, or foster homes to ensure that all the children were permanently safe and well and that the perpetrators were punished. There were some rescue stories, some stories with happy or at least tolerable endings—but there were too many stories with bad endings to make me very hopeful.

I don't think they ever found out who hurt the baby girl with the rope burns. There were suspicions, but nobody could prove them. She was taken away from her family initially, but I don't know where she is now. It is possible that she is back with them. She may be living with the person who hurt her.

I hope that she's okay. Her face haunts me, along with all the other faces of abused children that flash painfully through my mind in unguarded moments.

We have put men on the moon. We have built skyscrapers and incredibly complex computers. We have designed artificial hearts, eradicated polio, and cured thousands of people of cancer. Why can't we protect our children?

HEARTBEAT

The nurses called me to come see Angel a little after midnight. He was eight months old and had very bad asthma. They had given him some more medicine, but they weren't sure it had helped much. Would I come take a listen to his lungs?

The room was dark. I looked in Angel's crib; it was empty. Beside the crib was a cot where Angel's father lay with the baby on his chest. I knelt down and put my stethoscope on the baby's back.

"He sounds a little better," I said in Spanish. His father nodded.

I stayed there, looking at the two of them. His father smiled.

"At home, when they are sick, they all come sleep with me," he said in Spanish. "Sometimes you cannot see me, there are so many children on top of me."

He pointed to the crib. "Over there he gets scared," he said. "He does not know where I am."

His hand rested on the sleeping baby. "When he is here he can hear my heartbeat, and he knows where I am."

MELISSA'S
ILLNESS

She loved to play with my penlight.

It became a ritual with us. Whenever I would come near her, usually in the hallway as her parents wheeled her around in a little cart, propped up on pillows, I would hand her my penlight. She had learned how to press the little metal clip on the side to turn the light on; she would press it and smile at me. As long as she had my penlight, I could get close to her and listen to her chest, tap on her knees, do whatever I needed to do. It was our trade.

I met Melissa Dickerson in the late fall of 1989, during the neurology rotation I did while I was a second-year resident. Every fourth night when I was on call, along with taking care of the neurology patients in the hospital, I also was the neurology "consult," the person called if there was a patient anywhere in the hospital or in the emergency room who had a neurologic problem that the other doctors needed help with. Since I wasn't an expert in neurology, after I took the history and examined the patient I would call up the neurology chief resident and we would discuss the case and decide what should be done.

I still have the index card I used to take notes on when the intern called me from the emergency room about Melissa. "Fourteen-month-old," it reads. "Was walking, now not. Won't bear weight. Won't crawl. Has very stiff legs."

Melissa was whimpering in her mother's arms in one of the little examination rooms in the emergency room. Her mother, a tall, thin woman in her early thirties with long braided red hair, paced and rubbed Melissa's back. Melissa's father leaned against the wall. He wore a blue suit, his tie was undone, and his blond hair was tousled. He looked a few years younger than his wife.

I introduced myself. The mother kept pacing; the father came over and shook my hand.

"I'm Alan Dickerson," he said. "This is my wife, Rachel, and my daughter, Melissa." He paused. "Like I told the other doctor, we have an appointment with a neurologist here next week. I know we should probably just have waited for that appointment, but we were getting too worried."

There were two chairs in the room. "Would either of you like to sit down?" I asked.

"I'd rather stand, thanks," said Alan. Rachel shook her head. Melissa stopped whimpering; she rested her head on her mother's shoulder and closed her eyes. A blond curl fell across her face. I sat down.

"I know you've told the story to the other doctor, but it helps me to hear it straight from you. Would you mind?"

"We don't mind. Do you want to tell it, Rach?"

"No," said Rachel. "You do it better."

"Whatever. Like I told the other doctor, she was fine until right before her first birthday. More than fine, actually. She was great." He paused, looking at his daughter. "She was starting to walk, and she was into everything. When she crawled we practically had to run to keep up with her. She was strong, too—when anyone tried to take a toy away from her she gave them a good fight. She was so smart, too—she's always been smart. She can figure everyone and everything out."

He went over to the other chair. "Maybe I will sit down," he said. He sat down and leaned forward, his elbows resting on his knees.

"So anyway, around her first birthday she got sick. It was nothing at first—she had a fever and an ear infection. But the ear infection wouldn't go away, and, well, something was different. I mean, she'd had ear infections before, but they didn't affect her the way that one did. She just didn't get better even after the ear infection was gone. She didn't have a fever anymore, but she acted sick, kind of weak. Then we noticed she wasn't walking anymore.

"At first we thought she was just getting over being sick, but then she she stopped crawling, too. It was like she couldn't anymore. We would put her on the floor and she'd just lie there on her stomach."

"Did you take her to the pediatrician?" I asked.

Alan laughed, a brief, sarcastic laugh. "Sure, for all the good that did. He said that there was nothing wrong, that some kids walk later than others, and that we just needed to be patient. We tried to explain to him that the problem was that she had stopped walking, but he wouldn't listen."

I must have looked surprised.

"It's a big practice, and we always ended up seeing different people when Missy got sick, so the guy who is actually her doctor doesn't really know her very well. I don't know. We didn't want to think anything was wrong, and she was still as smart as ever, so we waited. But things got worse. We noticed that she couldn't really bend her legs right, and her arms seemed to be getting weaker—it was easy to pull a toy away from her. So we took her back to the pediatrician. He didn't seem too worried, but he said that something might be wrong, so he made an appointment for us with a neurologist."

He looked straight at me. His eyes were very blue and his gaze almost uncomfortably intent.

"We're not usually overanxious parents, honest. But we —or maybe I, I don't know—I couldn't wait until next week. There is something very wrong with my daughter."

His voice made me shiver. I looked away, looked down, scribbled some notes on the sheet of paper on my clipboard. He got up again and took off his jacket, which he draped over the chair. He went over to his wife and child.

"Here, let me hold her," he said. "You need a rest. You can answer the rest of the questions."

Carefully, Rachel gave Melissa to Alan. She whimpered a little in the transfer but then settled comfortably on her father's shoulder. She pushed the curls out of her face and watched me closely.

Rachel sat down on the edge of the stretcher. Her pale, freckled face was tired but beautiful. She had hazel eyes, a long, delicate nose, and full, rose-colored lips. Tendrils of hair fell softly around her face. She wore jeans and a plaid flannel shirt, but on her they looked elegant; she had a model's figure and grace.

I asked some questions about Melissa's medical history and developmental milestones. Besides the ear infections, she hadn't been sick, Rachel told me. I wrote down the ages at which she had done things like rolling over, sitting up, pulling to stand, saying words—all of them were normal. Rachel was earnest and serious as she spoke.

"Are there any illnesses that run in your family? Is there anyone who is retarded or has any kind of neurological problem?"

"Not in my family," said Rachel. Alan shook his head.

"Have you two been well? Have you had any medical problems?"

For the briefest of moments, I saw them exchange glances in a way that struck me as strange.

"We've been fine," Rachel said firmly.

I wondered if I should probe further, but I didn't know quite what to ask; I let it pass.

"What do the two of you do for work?"

"Alan is a manager in an advertising agency." She smiled. "He just got promoted."

"And you?"

"I'm a grad student in psychology, sort of. I took time off when Missy was born. I was planning on going back this fall, but since she was sick I decided to wait until next semester."

I put down my clipboard and picked up the purple zippered bag in which I kept my ophthalmoscope and other instruments.

"She's going to cry," said Rachel. "She hates doctors."

Melissa watched me as her father brought her over to the stretcher. She had his hair but her mother's hazel eyes, long eyelashes, and delicate features. She was thin and small. The hospital gown with its Disney characters looked huge on her.

I pulled my penlight out of my shirt pocket and pressed the clip to turn it on.

"Can you blow it out?" I asked her. She frowned at me.

"Like this," I said, blowing on the light and releasing the clip at the same time so that the light went out. Melissa still frowned at me.

"You try. Here." I held the penlight up to her mouth and turned it on. She looked at her parents, looked at me, pursed her lips, and blew. I let go of the clip so that the light went out as she blew. She stared at it with amazement.

"Again?" I asked. She nodded. We did it two more times, and then she smiled at me.

"Here," I said, and gave her the penlight. Her father put her down on the stretcher, and as she tried to figure out how to turn the light on, I examined her. Except for her thinness, her general exam was normal; her eyes, ears, and mouth were normal, her lungs and heart sounded fine, her abdominal exam didn't reveal a big liver or spleen or mass, her limbs were without any deformities, and her skin didn't show any rash or birthmark. Her neurologic exam, however, was very abnormal. As Alan had described, her arms and hands were weak, as were her trunk muscles. Without support, she didn't sit well. Her legs were very stiff; it was hard to bend them. Also, she wouldn't or couldn't bear weight on them. When I checked her reflexes they were extraordinarily brisk at her ankles and knees. They were brisk in her arms, too, but not as brisk as in her legs.

Melissa played diligently with the penlight, staring at it seriously. Finally, probably by accident, she grasped it in such a way that she pressed the clip and the light went on. She grinned and held it up, looking at her mother.

"Ite," she said.

"That's right, honey, it's a light," said Rachel, running her fingers through Melissa's hair.

I finished my exam. "Can I have my light back now, sweetie?"

Melissa frowned and turned toward Rachel.

"Give the doctor back her light, Missy," said Rachel.

Melissa turned back toward me and slowly, reluctantly, held out the penlight. I put it back in my pocket.

"Thank you very much," I said. "It was nice of you to give it back."

Melissa smiled, pleased with herself.

I excused myself to call the neurology chief resident.

When I told her the story and described the neurologic exam, she was worried. She wasn't sure what it was, but she thought we should admit Melissa to the hospital for further tests.

"We could probably wait for her appointment and do it all as an outpatient," she said, "but given how nervous the parents are and how, well, worrisome what you are describing to me is, I think we should admit her."

So we did; Alan and Rachel seemed relieved. I called the pediatrician, who seemed annoyed. "They are being over-anxious," he said. "They have an appointment to see a neurologist, but of course they just can't wait. These are really difficult parents." I said that we thought Melissa's story and physical examination were concerning and that we didn't blame them for being anxious, but he still seemed annoyed.

It was a Friday night, and the neurologist they had the appointment with wasn't available, so the next morning the chief resident and I presented Melissa's case to the neurologist doing rounds with us, an older man with a lot of experience. He examined Melissa, too, and then we sat down to talk about her.

"Whatever she's got," he said, "it isn't good." He thought it was probably one of the neurodegenerative disorders, diseases in which there is a breakdown of the neurologic system, most of them irreversible and many of them eventually fatal. However, he said, her symptoms and examination weren't classic for any of them. We went back, and the three of us sat with Alan and Rachel and asked lots of questions. We drew out a family tree, asked about the health and status of each family member, as many of the neurodegenerative diseases are inherited. We asked if there was any possible way there had been any intermarriage within or between their families, as this can sometimes bring out rare genetic disorders, but they said no. We went over the story of Melissa's illness and loss of abilities so many times, I think we all had every detail memorized. We asked every question possible— at least we thought we did.

We did so many tests. We did blood test after blood test, to the point that we made Melissa a little anemic. We did a spinal tap. We did urine tests. We took samples of her skin, muscles, and nerves for pathologists to study under the microscope. We did a CAT scan of her head. We did an MRI of her head and spinal cord. We did absolutely everything we could think of, looking for rare diseases, cancers, infections. We sent samples of blood and urine and tissues to laboratories all over the country. In looking back and thinking about the myriad tests we ran, it still amazes me that we never did the right one.

Not every result was normal. The level of protein in her cerebrospinal fluid was elevated, the MRI of her brain and spine showed some mild degeneration of the substance that coats nerves, and there were a few other small abnormalities in some of the other tests, but none of it seemed to fit together to give us a diagnosis. Like Alan, we knew something was very wrong with Melissa; we just couldn't figure out what it was.

Alan and Rachel were remarkably patient with us. I think they were happy that someone had finally listened to them and taken their concerns seriously.

Rachel was almost always there. She spent the nights on a cot next to Melissa's hospital crib and spent the days either sitting with Melissa during her tests or trying to find ways to amuse her. The hospital cart worked well. It was a wooden wagon with a back rest at one end that Rachel padded with a pillow. She would put Melissa in with some toys and off they would go, around the ward, to the cafeteria, to the lobby, wherever they were allowed to go as well as to a few places they weren't allowed but went anyway. Melissa loved it; she was shy but very curious, very interested in everyone and in everything around her.

Rachel never said very much. With Melissa, from a distance, she seemed animated. But whenever she noticed me watching or when I came to examine Melissa or talk with them, she would suddenly become subdued, and she rarely looked me in the eye. When I close my eyes now I can see her so clearly: her hair loosely braided, wearing faded jeans and a loose sweatshirt, sitting on the cot with Melissa on her lap. Melissa would lean against her, her hand on Rachel's arm, peacefully protected. They were extensions of one another, linked in tender touches, smiles, and an almost palpable trust.

There was something sad about Rachel, something different about her that I could never quite describe. There was something about the slow, soft way she moved, something about her seriousness and the way her eyes always looked away. She was very composed, always pleasant, very capable, wonderful with Melissa—but in the unguarded moments that I caught as I passed Melissa's room or turned a corner to find them in the hallway, Rachel always seemed so vulnerable and inexplicably fragile.

Alan came every day after work and spent all day on the weekend days. A couple of times he squeezed in with Rachel on the cot and spent the night, but mostly he went home to look after the dog and the house in Newton, the upper-middle-class suburb of Boston where they lived. He always had a lot of questions when he came in. He wanted to know the significance of each test and test result, and it was clear from his questions that every time we mentioned a possible diagnosis he went to the library and read everything he could find about it. I would try to sit down with them every day to keep them updated, although I didn't have much to say. Alan would sit next to Rachel, his body close to hers and his arm around her as we spoke. If Melissa fussed, he would pick her up and hold her close, too. His voice, his hands, his whole body language, were fiercely protective.

Once when I was playing with Melissa I looked up and saw Alan watching Rachel, who was talking on the phone. He looked at her with longing and with something else—it was as if he were afraid for her, or of her, I'm not sure.

In the midst of the tests, Melissa caught a cold. Her parents were worried, but I wasn't. She had a runny nose and a cough, and she was breathing a little fast, but it didn't seem serious, and given how serious her neurologic problems were, I didn't pay much attention to it.

After about ten days we discharged Melissa from the hospital. She still had the cold, but it hadn't gotten worse, nor had her neurologic symptoms. As Melissa played with my penlight, I explained to Alan and Rachel that although we didn't have a diagnosis we felt sure that something would show up in the tests we had sent to the outside laboratories, that somehow we would figure out what was going on with Melissa. I told them that we had arranged for them to have an appointment in one week with the neurologist they were originally supposed to see, who had been following and guiding Melissa's workup in the hospital. I wished them luck and told them I had enjoyed getting to know them.

I stood up. Melissa looked up at me, holding the penlight. She knew this was when she had to give it back.

I smiled. "That's okay, honey. You can keep it. I have more."

Melissa understood perfectly. She grinned, turned the light on, and turned to Rachel.

"Mine," she said.

"That's right, Missy," said Rachel. "It's yours now."

Four or five days after Melissa was discharged Alan paged me. He sounded upset.

"I'm sorry to bother you," he said, "but Missy's sick and I didn't know who to call."

I was about to ask why he hadn't called their pediatrician when he said, "We don't want to go back to her old pediatrician."

That was understandable, I thought, given all that had happened.

"We've got some names of other pediatricians, but we haven't made an appointment with any of them, so none of them know her at all."

"What's going on?"

"You know that cold she had in the hospital?"

"Yes?"

"She's really sick with it now. She's got a fever, and all she does is cough—it kept her up all last night. Her nose is all stuffed up, and she really seems to be having trouble breathing. I stayed home from work today, and we've been trying to get her to eat something, but she won't. She's barely even drinking—I think it's because she's having so much trouble breathing."

"It sounds like she needs to come to the emergency room. Can you bring her now?"

"Sure. We'll come right over."

I called the emergency room to let them know she was coming and tell them what I knew about her. As I got off the phone I wondered if this cold could have something to do with her neurologic problems. No, probably not, I thought.

When she arrived she was indeed very sick and was admitted to the hospital. She was admitted to a medical floor, not the neurology floor, so I wasn't her resident anymore. She was diagnosed as having RSV, respiratory synctial virus, an illness that causes bad cold symptoms. Small infants can get very sick with this virus, but it was a little strange that a child of Melissa's age was so sick, especially since she didn't have any underlying problems with her lungs or her immune system that we knew of.

I went by to see her the next morning. She was lying very still in the crib, breathing rapidly. She was pale and seemed thinner. I was startled by how sick she looked.

"Where are her parents?" I asked the nurse.

"I sent them home. They looked like they hadn't slept in days. They spent all last night just staring at her."

Looking at Melissa, I understood why. How had she gotten so sick so quickly? What had we missed?

"I don't like the looks of her," said the nurse, taking an oxygen mask off the wall and putting it over Melissa's face as she turned on the oxygen. "Maybe this will make her a little more comfortable."

I left, feeling confused and guilty. Maybe we shouldn't have discharged her when we did, I thought. But it was just a cold, and she hadn't seemed that sick.

I started a new rotation the next day, in the neonatal intensive care unit at Brigham and Women's Hospital. Although the hospital is right next to Children's, I found it difficult to get over to visit Melissa and her parents; it was a demanding rotation with little free time. It was about three days before I went to see Melissa again, and when I went to the ward she wasn't there.

I asked one of the nurses where she was.

"Oh, she's in the ICU."

"The intensive care unit? What happened?"

"She got really sick a couple of nights ago, and they had to intubate her. I hear she's not doing so well over there."

I went over to the ICU. Melissa was indeed intubated, on a ventilator that was breathing for her. Medications ran through intravenous lines into her bloodstream. Monitors on the shelf above her bed continuously measured her heart rate, blood pressure, and oxygen saturation. Heavily sedated, she didn't move at all. Rachel sat on a stool next to the bed, holding Melissa's hand and whispering to her. Alan was pacing.

I wasn't sure what to say. They didn't seem to want to talk anyway. Rachel acknowledged my presence with a nod and went back to whispering to Melissa. I couldn't really hear her, but at one point I thought I heard her say, "You have to get better, honey, you just have to." She leaned over the bed as if she wanted to climb in next to Melissa.

I asked Alan if they had gotten any results back from the tests we had sent, if anyone had any more ideas about Melissa's diagnosis. He shook his head.

"Nobody seems to know anything," he said. "I've stopped asking questions—it's too depressing to keep hearing everyone say they don't know."

I reached over and touched his arm. "We'll figure it out, I know we will."

He shrugged and looked over at Melissa and Rachel. "God, I hope so."

Over the next week Melissa's condition grew steadily worse. She required more and more help from the ventilator to breathe. Her lungs were in terrible shape. It seemed as if she had another infection there besides the RSV. More test results came back, but all of them were normal, knocking one diagnosis after another off our list of possibilities. And we still couldn't explain why she was so sick with the lung infections.

I came by the ICU late one evening on my way home. I hadn't been there in a couple of days, and something seemed different, something about the way Alan and Rachel and Melissa's nurse were acting. I could see it from a distance. The ICU junior resident was sitting in the glassed-in doctor's room, looking up lab values on the computer. I ducked in before Alan or Rachel saw me and sat on the chair next to him.

"What's up with Dickerson?"

He turned. "Oh," he said. "You didn't hear?" He was very serious.

"I've been over at the Brigham. What is it?"

He leaned closer to me. "She's HIV positive."

I was stunned. "She has AIDS?"

"Yes."

So it was part of the same thing, her neurologic problems and her cold. The virus that causes AIDS makes it very hard for the body to fight infections. That's why she had gotten so sick with RSV.

"How?"

"How'd she get it? Mom was transfused nine years ago. No other risk factors, so probably that was it. They're very funny about talking about it—I think it was a suicide attempt."

We'd never asked Rachel about transfusions. As I thought about it, I realized there were lots of things we never asked her. I remembered the exchange of glances in the emergency room.

"So all the neurological stuff—it's AIDS?"

"Apparently so. None of the neurologists have seen anything like it before. They see neurological stuff with AIDS, of course, but not like this. I think one of them found a case report that was similar, but that's it."

"So Mom—"

"Is positive, too. Yeah. We had her seen by an internist yesterday—she's actually not in great shape. Hopefully they can get her on some AZT."

So the thinness, the fragility . . .

"And Dad?"

"Negative."

"How did you guys think of testing for HIV?"

"There was just something weird about how sick the kid was with RSV. It wasn't right. It didn't make sense—unless there was something else going on with her." He got up. "I need to go change an IV in one of the other kids. You gonna talk to the parents?"

I nodded. He left.

Melissa had AIDS. Why hadn't we thought of it while she was on the neurology service? Maybe the neurologists hadn't seen findings like hers in children with AIDS, but AIDS was such a new disease that we couldn't possibly know what we might expect. In other patients, when symptoms and signs weren't explainable, we often invoked AIDS at least as a possible contributing factor. Why had nobody even mentioned AIDS in Melissa's case?

Was it because her problem was just neurologic except for the cold that wasn't so bad at the time? Maybe. But it wasn't uncommon for AIDS to present with neurologic symptoms alone. This had been seen in adults. Was it because she was a blond little girl born to educated, upper-middle-class parents? I didn't like to think so, but maybe it was true.

I got up and went out into the open hallway leading to Melissa's bed space. Alan was pacing. He looked up and saw me. He walked over to me; I gave him a hug.

"I'm really sorry," I said.

He let go of me and leaned against the wall. "I just can't believe it," he said. "My wife and my daughter have AIDS. Shit, AIDS isn't something that happens to people like us. AIDS is what happens to drug addicts and gays and people like that. Not us." He looked away and bit his lip.

I leaned against the wall, too. "What happened to Rachel?"

He looked back at the bed space where Rachel sat near Melissa.

"Not here," he said. "Is there any place where she wouldn't hear?"

"How about there?" I pointed to the doctor's room. He looked back again and then nodded.

We went in and he sat on one of the orange vinyl armchairs. I sat on a chair facing him. He leaned forward, rubbing the sides of his head.

"Don't talk to Rachel about this, okay?" he said. "It really doesn't matter, anyway—the bottom line is that she got transfused, and it doesn't matter why. But I feel like telling this to someone. Maybe I want to defend her, I don't know."

He leaned back on the chair for a moment, then leaned forward again. He looked anxious and uncomfortable.

"Rachel was married before. She was young, she didn't get along with her parents, she dropped out of college—you get the picture. So she married this guy who seemed great—handsome, charming, money, the works. Turns out he's an alcoholic, and when he got drunk he got mean. Used to beat her up all the time. She told him she wanted a divorce, but he said that if she tried, he'd kill her. She believed him, and from what she's told me about him I'd believe him, too."

He paused for a moment, his hands over his face. "She told me she felt like she had no way out and that she couldn't live that way anymore. So she cut her wrists. It was a long time before her husband found her, and by then she had bled so much that they had to transfuse her to save her life."

And at that time they weren't testing the blood supply for HIV.

"What happened to the husband?"

"He got himself killed in a car accident a few months later. He was driving drunk."

Alan got up and paced back and forth in the little room. "When I met her she was still a mess. But things had really been working out. I think I've been good for her, and she was back in school. Every once in a while she'd bring it up, and I'd say, 'Rachel, don't even think about that stuff, it's all in the past and it can't hurt you now.' God, was I wrong." He looked away, and his eyes filled with tears.

"Look, don't tell people about this, okay?" he said. "It was a really bad time in Rachel's life, and she doesn't like people to know about it. But please tell people it wasn't her fault."

"I will."

He went back to the bed space. I sat there for a couple of seconds and then followed him.

Rachel was standing next to Melissa, stroking her hair. Melissa lay with her eyes closed, the endotracheal tube going through her nostril into her windpipe. She was even paler than before, and her face was bloated. Her only movement was the rising and falling of her chest with each breath given by the ventilator. I glanced at her flow sheet; her numbers looked very bad. She was going to die.

I put my arm around Rachel's shoulders, but she resisted me, moving closer to Melissa. Leave me alone with my baby, she seemed to be saying. Go away. Alan stood at the foot of the bed, staring at the two of them.

I went to the other side of the bed and touched Melissa's hand. "Good-bye, honey," I said under my breath.

Rachel looked over at me. Her face was blank. Her eyes were looking into mine for the first time, but I don't think she really saw me. She looked right through me; she was somewhere else. She was somewhere else with her baby.

I took a step back and nodded good-bye to Alan and

Rachel. As I turned to leave, something on the bedside table caught my eye.

It was my penlight.

There was nothing that could be done. Melissa Dickerson died the following morning of respiratory failure caused by overwhelming lung infection, a complication of AIDS.

THE MOMENT
OF BIRTH

*T*here is so much in that moment, that beginning, ending, in-between moment of actual birth, as the baby emerges from his home in the womb into the outside and away from the connections that have kept him alive. It is a moment when breaths are held and hearts quicken as those present wait to see if the baby will breathe and take on his separateness.

In most births it is not a frightening moment. In most births all present are confident that the breath will be taken and the child will be vigorous, because the woman is healthy, the pregnancy has gone well, and labor has proceeded smoothly and predictably. But in some births there is less confidence and it is frightening.

I leaned against the cement wall of the delivery room, waiting. I wore a yellow gown over my scrubs, but still I shivered; the room was cold. My hair was tucked under a paper cap, I wore paper covers over my sneakers and a surgical mask across my mouth and nose. The room was being converted into an operating room.

It didn't take many changes to convert it. It was already so clean and bare that it echoed in the corners. Bright fluorescent lights shone from the high ceiling. To make it an operating room, everyone put on masks and one of the nurses brought out surgical instruments to lay on the draped metal tables.

The triage nurse from the neonatal intensive care unit, Angela, stood next to me. She was dressed as I was, and she was waiting, too. Every time I went to a delivery, a triage nurse came with me, which was good. They had all been to many more deliveries than I, and their experience was very helpful. Some were reticent with advice; some told me exactly what to do, with condescending disdain, whether I asked them for help or not. Angela was somewhere in between. She was quick and capable, always pleasant, and she worked independently while working with me. I liked being on call with her.

The neonatal intensive care unit, or NICU, is right next to Labor and Delivery at the Brigham and Women's Hospital. A set of swinging doors separates the entrance area of the NICU and the long gray hallway lined with big sinks where the obstetricians wash their hands before and after deliveries. The rooms along this hallway were called delivery rooms, but they could become operating rooms at a moment's notice to do a cesarean section or whatever surgery was necessary. As you walked down the hallway and peered through the small windows in the doors, it felt much more like a surgical suite than a place where babies were born.

Past the delivery rooms, through another set of automated swinging doors, were the labor rooms and the birthing rooms where uncomplicated deliveries took place. They were smaller and cozier, with dimmer lighting and wallpapered

walls. They were farther from the NICU, but the pediatricians were less often needed in those rooms.

*T*hey called us early to this delivery—too
early, I thought. The woman was just being brought into the
room on a stretcher. It would be a while before the baby
was out, but Angela and I really had no choice but to wait.
If we left, we might not get back there fast enough. Every
second could be crucial.

I couldn't get used to always trying to get to a delivery
fast enough. It put me on edge. I knew what to do in almost
any medical situation with a newborn; we had been carefully
trained. But rushing made it hard for me to think clearly or
plan. It flustered me, made me unsure.

I spent my days and nights on call running from one
delivery to another. That was my job as the pediatric resident
on call for deliveries. When Labor and Delivery called the
NICU, an overhead bell went off simultaneously as the
phone rang, alerting me. As soon as I heard the bell I was
on my feet, reaching for the metal toolbox filled with resuscitation equipment and medicines. I wore a beeper, but most
of the time the secretary just yelled for me. She would bark
out instructions loudly in no particular direction, expecting
me and the triage nurse to hear. She would tell us where to
go and the reason we were going, although the information
was usually minimal. We never really knew how serious
something was going to be until we got there. Some of the
pediatric residents found this exciting. I didn't. If there was
a possibility that I was going to have to save a life, I preferred
to know ahead of time.

The triage nurse and I would run to the cart by the swinging doors for gloves and fresh paper caps. I usually kept my

sneakers covered and left a mask hanging around my neck so it could be quickly pulled up and tied. It saved time.

They transferred the woman off the stretcher onto the table in the middle of the room. She was small; her arms and legs looked tiny and thin, completely out of proportion to her huge belly. Her brown hair was long and curly and tangled. Her face was the only uncovered face in the room, which drew attention to it immediately. She was pale, with large round eyes that darted around the room like those of a frightened animal. She wore only a short hospital gown, and she shivered in the cold room. She reached down to touch her belly, but one of the obstetrical nurses took her hand away and put a probe on one of her fingers to measure the oxygen saturation in her blood. There was nobody with her. They don't admit husbands or family or friends when they do an emergency C-section.

"Stat C-section for fetal distress," was what the secretary told us when Labor and Delivery called about this delivery. When we arrived at the room, the nurse gave us the rest of the story. The woman was twenty-nine years old, it was her first pregnancy, and it had been uncomplicated. A prenatal ultrasound had shown the baby to be a boy without any major birth defects. She had gone into labor a few days before her due date, in a very normal and usual way, and for the first few hours things seemed to be progressing well. Then, for some reason, things got stuck; the baby just wouldn't come out. Then the monitors that had been wrapped around the woman's belly to measure the baby's heart rate and contractions began to show the baby's heart rate dropping down with each contraction. This was a bad sign. It meant that the baby was in trouble.

They tried various maneuvers to get the baby to drop

down to where they could reach him with forceps, but nothing worked. The heart rate was dropping lower and staying low longer. The obstetrician decided that it was time for an emergency C-section.

A pediatrician wasn't called to every delivery, of course. We were called only when there was concern about the baby. Sometimes the concern was well defined, such as prematurity or the presence of birth defects on a prenatal ultrasound. A lot of the time, though, the concern was not so clear; those were the "fetal distress" calls. The obstetricians knew something wasn't right, they knew the baby was in trouble, but they didn't know exactly why.

Most of the time, when they called us for fetal distress, the babies actually needed very little help. The obstetricians handed the baby over to us all wet and slippery. The baby was usually bluish, limp, and not crying. They laid him on blankets on the warming table under the lights, and the triage nurse and I quickly gathered up the edges of the blankets and dried him vigorously. We used a bulb syringe to suck out amniotic fluid from the baby's mouth and nose. The triage nurse usually did more than I; she was more expert at these things. Her hands moved quickly and confidently around the baby, encouraging and coaxing him into his new life.

Usually, somehow, that was all we needed to do. In most births, nature took care of the babies, and we just watched. With the drying and stimulation the baby would usually start to cry, and with those deep breaths he would become pink and his arms and legs would draw up close to his body with the nice muscle tone we like to see in newborn babies. As his cries filled the room, everyone would relax. It can be such music, a baby's first cry.

But sometimes we needed to do more, and that possibility always frightened me.

One of the obstetrical nurses gathered the woman's curls up under a cap like mine. The woman looked up at her, biting her lip. The anesthesiologist leaned over the woman and began to talk to her softly. He was tall and thin, and he wore wire-rimmed glasses over his mask. His movements were easy, gentle, reassuring.

I couldn't make out everything he was saying. He seemed to be explaining what he was going to do and what she was going to feel. Then he turned and pointed at me.

"That's the pediatrician," he said in a louder but still gentle voice. "She's here in case the baby needs any help when he's born. She'll take good care of him."

The woman stared at me with confused and imploring eyes. I nodded at her; she nodded back. I wished the anesthesiologist hadn't said anything. She's trusting me with her baby now, I thought. I hope I deserve it.

There were two obstetricians in the room, a short one and a tall one. I knew the short one; he was very experienced, with an excellent reputation, although people said he was often gruff with his patients. The tall one seemed young, a little unsure. He was probably an obstetrical resident called in to assist.

One of the nurses looked at the baby's heart rate tracing and said something about the rate still being low.

"Everything's going to be fine, Linda," said the short obstetrician in a voice that was maybe a little too loud. "We're going to put you to sleep now, and when you wake up we'll have a beautiful baby to show you."

*I*f the father was in the room, we invited him over once the baby was pink and vigorous. We usually had to invite them over. They hung behind, afraid of being in the way. We'd bring over the father and show him his baby, counting the fingers and toes, commenting on the hair or eyes or nose. There was always something we could say resembled the father. "What's his name?" we'd ask, and proudly the father would tell us as he stared with wonderment and incredulity at the tiny human being that was his child. Even though the father had spent months watching the mother's belly grow and feeling the kicks with his hands, I don't think the baby was ever real to him until that moment.

"You can touch him if you'd like," we'd say, and the father would reach out slowly, gingerly, with his finger, touching the baby's hand. Almost always, the tiny fingers would close around his. I never got tired of watching that moment, of watching the father's face shine.

Then the triage nurse would swaddle the baby, wrapping him up tightly in a clean blanket like a little papoose, and bring him over to the mother, unless she was completely anesthetized or unstable. The mothers were full of wonderment, too, but theirs was different. They were meeting outside the child they had known inside, the child who had been real to them, just unseen. They were less tentative; they touched with more confidence.

*T*he anesthesiologist injected something into the intravenous catheter in the woman's arm, and within a couple of minutes her eyes were closing. When she was asleep he opened her mouth wide with a laryngoscope and inserted a breathing tube into her windpipe, through which he could control her breathing and give her more anesthetic. They don't like to use general anesthesia when delivering babies. Inevitably the baby absorbs some of the anesthetic before he is born and comes out sleepy and lethargic. In an emergency, though, there are fewer choices. General anesthesia is quick.

"All set here," he said.

The obstetrician looked at the resident. "Ready?" he asked. The resident nodded.

They cleaned the woman's belly with Betadine and laid blue sterile cloths around it. They worked quickly. The short obstetrician asked for a scalpel. The room was very quiet; the only sound was the woman's heart monitor, counting off her heartbeat in a muted tone.

He cut through the skin across her lower abdomen; there was a line of blood. Rapidly he cut deeper, through the fat and muscle. The resident used retractors to pull open the incision.

"Okay, there's the uterus," said the obstetrician. The room grew even quieter.

He asked for a new scalpel and opened the uterus. There was a rush of clear fluid, which the scrub nurse quickly cleared away with a suction catheter. The resident moved the retractors so that they pulled open the uterine incision, and the obstetrician reached inside.

He frowned, twisting his arm around slightly. "Nuchal cord," he said.

This meant that the umbilical cord was wrapped around the baby's neck. I felt some relief. This could easily have caused the drops in the baby's heart rate, and it was easy to fix. The cord just had to be unwrapped. I hoped it was the only problem the baby had.

He worked at something within the uterus for a few

seconds—I assumed he was taking the cord off the baby's neck—and then he put both hands inside and pulled, hard. Soon the head emerged above the incision. I couldn't really see much, because the resident was standing in my way.

I heard the resident suction out the baby's mouth and nose with a bulb syringe. There was no cry. Then the obstetrician pulled the rest of the baby out of the uterus. Nobody said anything, which worried me. Usually someone says something when a baby is born. They quickly clamped the cord in two places and cut between the clamps. Then the resident brought the baby over to Angela and me, urgently, laying him on the warming table in front of us.

*I*t was that first, in-between, uncertain moment that I dreaded. The obstetricians did their job, and then it was my turn, my responsibility to keep the new life going and make it stronger. Even though I had the skills and equipment and medicines to do it, even though nature usually did most of the work, it was still overwhelming.

The baby boy was small, although not much smaller than average, with lots of black hair matted with blood and amniotic fluid. He didn't cry; he wasn't breathing. He was very blue, and he lay limp and motionless under the lights, his eyes closed.

This baby is barely alive, I thought. I remembered the woman's eyes as she stared at me.

Angela began to rub the baby vigorously with the blanket. I reached for the bulb syringe and cleared his mouth and nose of fluid and mucus. There wasn't much there, but I was hoping it would bother him enough to make him cry. He didn't cry; all he did was take a couple of gasping breaths. Angela reached over for the newborn-size oxygen mask and held it over the baby's face.

I did a quick examination of the baby. There were no deformities to suggest birth defects. He was completely limp and unresponsive. I listened with my stethoscope. With the rare breaths he was taking, it sounded as though his lungs still had fluid in them. He didn't have a heart murmur, but his heart rate was slower than it should have been. In newborn babies, that's usually caused by lack of oxygen.

"Heart rate's about eighty," I said to Angela. "Lungs sound horrible."

Angela pushed the mask tighter over the baby's mouth and nose and gave the baby breaths by pushing on the bag attached to the mask. If we could open up his lungs a little, get some more oxygen into him, maybe he would start breathing on his own.

The obstetricians were working on delivering the placenta, but they were watching us silently. The anesthesiologist stared at us, his hand resting on the sleeping woman's shoulder. The obstetrical nurse stood a few feet from the warming table, her arms crossed in front of her, her forehead creased in a nervous frown.

"Let's see what he'll do," I said. Angela took off the mask, and the two of us looked down at the baby.

He did nothing. He lay there just as limp and almost as blue despite the oxygen. He didn't breathe at all. I checked his heart rate.

"Fifty," I said.

Quickly Angela put the mask back on, and I began to do chest compressions, pressing down on the baby's chest with my fingers, trying to pump blood out of the baby's heart into his body.

We were fighting nature this time. If we let nature take its course, the baby would die. What was going on? It could just be the nuchal cord, but that alone didn't usually make a baby look this bad. Maybe it was the anesthesia; although they got the baby out pretty quickly after the woman was asleep, even a little bit in the baby's system, in combination with the nuchal cord, could do this. But was I missing something? Did the baby have some sort of severe infection? Was there a lung problem or heart problem that the ultrasound hadn't picked up? The woman's eyes flashed through my mind again and again.

"Stop CPR," I said. "Let's check."

The baby's color was a little better, but that was probably because of the oxygen and chest compressions. He took a couple of breaths, but they were not good ones. Angela checked his heart rate by feeling the pulse in the stump of the umbilical cord.

"Ninety," she said.

That was better, but it needed to be at least over a hundred.

"Maybe you should intubate," said Angela.

She was right. Putting a breathing tube down would allow us to get oxygen into the lungs more easily and efficiently. With the mask we were blowing a lot into the stomach. A tube would give us more control.

But my stomach sank when she said it. The fact that we needed to intubate just reinforced the seriousness of this moment. The baby's life was still very much in danger. Also, intubation could be difficult. It was easy to miss the windpipe and slip the tube into the esophagus instead. What if I couldn't do it?

I nodded to Angela. She put the mask back on and gave the baby some more breaths while I got a laryngoscope and an endotracheal tube out of the resuscitation box.

She took off the mask. I put the laryngoscope into the baby's mouth, pushing back the tongue. I held the tube in my other hand, the tip in the baby's mouth. As Angela pushed down slightly on the baby's neck I looked for the vocal cords, the entrance into the windpipe.

"Heart rate's dropping," Angela said quietly.

Suddenly the vocal cords came into view, and I pushed the tube forward, praying it would go in the right place.

"I think you're in," said Angela. "I felt it."

I held the tube carefully in place. Angela quickly took the mask off the oxygen bag and attached the bag to the tube. She put on her stethoscope and listened to each side of the baby's chest as she pushed some oxygen through the tube.

"It's in," she said. "Heart rate's coming up, too." I realized I had been holding my breath, and I let it out, still holding tightly to the tube.

She taped the tube to the baby's face, and I let go. I held the bag and gave the baby regular breaths through the tube, watching the chest rise and fall much better than it had before. Angela listened with her stethoscope.

"Hundred and ten or so. Lungs are opening up." She smiled at me. "How about we get out of here?"

"Sure," I said. Back in the NICU there were neonatologists, specialists in the care of newborns. I was quite ready to turn over to them the responsibility for this baby.

Angela looked up at the obstetrical nurse, who was still close by and watching. "Do me a favor," she said. "Could you go get the incubator that's down by the doors?" The nurse nodded and scurried out of the room.

While Angela called the NICU to tell them we were coming, I kept giving the baby breaths. He was much pinker now, and he was starting to get some muscle tone. His arms and legs were held slightly bent instead of being limp at his sides. With my free hand I reached over and pinched his foot; he pulled it away. He didn't do it as quickly or strongly as I would have liked, but at least he was responding.

"How are things going over there?" the short obstetrician asked loudly, looking up from sewing the woman's abdomen.

I was glad he had waited to ask. "Better," I said. "Much better."

The obstetrical nurse brought in the incubator, and Angela and I transferred the baby inside, switching over to the incubator's oxygen supply and slipping the bag through one of the armholes as we closed up the sides.

"The father is in the waiting room," said the obstetrical nurse. "I know you don't have time now, but when you can—"

I nodded as we pushed the incubator out of the room. We moved quickly and wordlessly down the corridor that seemed eternally long, giving the baby breaths and watching him through the glass. Finally we were through the swinging doors, and the secretary was pointing us into one of the rooms.

Two neonatologists, a nurse, and a respiratory therapist were waiting for us. Suddenly there were many hands, reaching for the baby, bringing him to a brightly lit warming table, hooking up the tube to a respirator, attaching monitors to his chest, putting an intravenous catheter into his hand. I stepped back and watched the hands as they moved around and over and on the baby so deftly, so expertly. I listened to the tones of the monitors and the light, quick conversation among the nurse, the neonatologists, and the respiratory therapist, these people so used to working with tiny and tenuous lives, so comfortable with the possibility of a crisis or even death. I knew I could never be that way.

I gave my sign-out to the intern working in the room, telling her what I knew about the prenatal history and summarizing what had happened after the delivery. I stayed for a while, watching. The baby's vital signs stabilized. His breathing became more regular. There was nothing seriously wrong with him, no infection or other problem; it just had been the nuchal cord and the anesthesia. The combination had been enough to nearly kill him, but we had done what we needed to do, and he was going to be okay.

Angela came up behind me, tapping me on the shoulder. "Don't forget the dad," she said.

"Oh, yeah," I said, startled, and went back through the doors, along the corridor, through the next set of doors, and past the labor rooms into the waiting room. I pulled off my cap and ran my fingers through my hair.

As I got there I realized I had forgotten the woman's last name, but I knew the father immediately. He was dressed in scrubs, walking back and forth across the room with slow but agitated steps. He was tall, with a brown mustache, and he clasped and unclasped his big hands in front of him.

I caught his eye. "I'm Dr. McCarthy, from Pediatrics," I said.

He stopped and looked full at me, his eyes expectant and frightened.

"Your son—he's going to be okay," I said.

He brought his hands to his face. "Oh, thank God," he said softly.

"You can come see him, if you'd like."

He nodded, and I led him back past the labor rooms into the corridor.

"The nurse said my wife's okay," he said. It sounded like a question.

"They were still sewing her up when I left," I said. "Everything seemed fine." It was a vague answer, but he seemed reassured.

As we walked I told him what had happened and what we'd done, but I don't think he was listening. He stared ahead, walking quickly and deliberately at my side.

The swinging doors opened in front of us, and I brought him into the room where we'd brought the baby. He paused in the entrance, blinking as he adjusted to the dim lighting, looking around at the warming tables and incubators and monitors lining the walls of the little room.

"Over there," I said, pointing to the warming table in the corner. The neonatologist and the nurse were standing by the table, smiling, and they motioned him over.

The breathing tube was out. The baby didn't need it anymore; he was breathing well on his own. His blue eyes were open, squinting at the light above him, and his small arms reached up.

The father approached the table tentatively and looked down at the baby.

"He's very handsome," said the nurse. "Does he have a name?"

The father smiled. "His name is Andrew," he said. "Andrew Jacob."

"Andrew is going to be fine," she said. "He just had a rough start."

The father reached over carefully, slowly, and touched the baby's hand with his index finger. Immediately the baby's fingers closed tightly around his finger, and the in-between, uncertain moment passed.

JONNY

Jonny was born prematurely, at twenty-six weeks. His lungs were very immature, and for several months he was dependent on the ventilator for his breathing. Many times his lungs collapsed or got infected, making it very hard to get oxygen into his blood. Because of this, his brain was damaged, and he had seizures. He developed necrotizing enterocolitis, an intestinal problem common in premature babies, and had to have a large section of his intestine removed.

He nearly died many times, but thanks to medical science, advanced technology, and fate, he survived. Eventually he was weaned from the ventilator, but he couldn't be weaned from oxygen and constantly wore tubing that blew oxygen into his nose. His seizures couldn't be stopped entirely, but with lots of medications they became less frequent. His intestines healed, but he had very little of them left to digest food with. He had to be fed a specially made formula very slowly, via a tube that the surgeons put into his stomach through his abdominal wall.

I didn't know him then, but I knew babies like him. Their lives started out as one crisis after another, daily near misses with death. Those kinds of situations galvanize doctors, and tremendous thought, energy, and skill was invested in keeping babies such as Jonny alive. Rarely did we think about what lay ahead for them. We couldn't let death beat us. As the babies' conditions stabilized they were moved off to corners of the unit, and we paid little attention to them, although we grew used to having them there and felt a sort of distracted fondness for them.

*J*onny got too old to be in the newborn intensive care unit and was transferred to the infant ward, which is where I met him. He lived there in his crib or infant seat, always attached to oxygen. He required frequent suctioning of his windpipe and medications to help him breathe.

His mother was a young, unsophisticated woman. She was small and slight, with long brown hair. She wore dresses that were too big, and she looked down when you spoke to her. I never met his father; I'm not sure he even knew Jonny had been born. I heard that at first Jonny's mother came to visit every day, but by the time he went to the infant ward it was more like once a week. The technology involved in his daily life must have been overwhelming for her. It probably frightened her to hold him or be alone with him, thinking that his tubes might come dislodged or one of his monitor alarms would go off or that, somehow, she might hurt him. Some mothers adapt to this and become almost nurselike, comfortable with the machines and the medicines. Some, like Jonny's mother, grow sad and frustrated and end up staying away.

The nurses did their best to make Jonny's life pleasant. They hung pictures and placed bright toys in his crib. They played with him whenever they could, brought him and his oxygen tank into their conference room, and held him on their laps while they wrote their notes or "gave report." But they had other patients to take care of, and Jonny spent the majority of his waking hours alone in his crib or sitting on his seat in the hallway.

I used to wonder what it was like to sit in that seat. They sat him across from the front desk of the ward so people were always passing by: people in white coats, nurses in scrub pants or dresses, parents and visitors and children. Occasionally people would stop to talk to him, but mostly it must have been a relatively uninteresting parade. There was plenty of noise: monitor alarms going off, overhead pages, phones ringing, and lots of voices. Sometimes the nurses would put other patients on seats near him, but rarely did any of them interact with him. They were mostly children who, like Jonny, had some degree of brain damage along with their chronic health problems. They didn't really interact with anyone; they all just sat there on their seats and watched the world of the ward go by.

Days and weeks and months passed. Jonny had his first birthday, and the nurses threw him a party. More months passed. He was small for his age but chubby; the steroids he needed every day to help his lungs made his cheeks full and his belly round. He had blond hair that the nurses kept neatly trimmed and small blue eyes that didn't see very well because of retinal damage, another common complication of being a sick premature baby.

It was hard to know the extent of his brain damage. His motor skills were very delayed. He was able to sit and grasp things, but he was never able to crawl or stand or do anything else. He never spoke; he barely made noise.

But he smiled sometimes, for instance when his favorite nurses tickled him or made silly faces at him, and he definitely had reactions and expressions that were subtle but obvious if you knew him well enough. The nurses were convinced that he knew and understood more than we realized. It may have been true. It may have been that he used up so much of his energy trying to breathe that he couldn't show us what he knew.

I wonder if he was lonely or bored or if he missed his mother. I wonder if there was something he wanted that we never knew, or if he was happy in his little world.

I wonder what they all thought, all those children who sat in hallways and cribs, children who were alive only because heroic measures had been taken and were still being taken, who had uncertain and probably limited futures, who didn't take part in the world in any way we could really understand.

It wasn't so bad when the families adapted, when they stayed with them in the hospital or outfitted rooms where they lived so that they could take the children home sometimes. Those children still had uncertain and limited futures, but they had love and a family, and there is not much else I could wish for any child. It was the ones whose parents couldn't adapt or the ones whose medical needs prevented them from ever leaving a hospital or institution that made me feel sad and confused about how some medical decisions are made.

*T*he lung damage Jonny had was extensive and severe, and whenever he caught a cold or just got tired, he had to be transferred to the intensive care unit because he required a ventilator to breathe or constant nursing care.

These trips were frequent, and each time there was some doubt as to whether he would live.

But somehow he did. The doctors and nurses in the intensive care unit worked very hard to save him, and thanks to their efforts, as well as that same advanced technology and fate, he survived.

There were constant plans, constant arrangements, being made for the day when he would be ready to leave the hospital and go home. He did go home once, with lots of equipment and visiting nurses twenty-four hours a day, but in less than a week his breathing deteriorated and he needed to come back to the hospital.

It was more of a surprise than it should have been when Jonny died shortly before his second birthday. We should have known, and we probably did, that his lungs would eventually give out.

One could argue that given the slim chance of his eventual survival, we shouldn't have saved him all those other times. His care, and the care of children like him, cost hundreds of thousands of dollars; perhaps it was money that could have been better used to buy medicines for poor children or pay for a lifesaving organ transplant.

One could argue, too, that it wasn't kind to keep saving him because he didn't have much of a life, sitting in the hallway or lying in the intensive care unit. That's hard to say, though. Jonny didn't know anything else; to him it must have felt normal and become his home. He may very well have been happy.

Once heroic measures have been taken for a child, it's hard to stop taking them. It's as if we feel a commitment, a responsibility, or perhaps an unwillingness to consider the possibility that we might have been wrong.

It's especially hard when we think there's even a glimmer of hope that the child will get better. We saw that glimmer with Jonny, although it was very faint. It was hard, too, to have perspective when we were in the middle of something. Besides, Jonny had been with us for so long that we had come to love him.

It almost always feels better and more right to save a life than to let one end, but sometimes it isn't better or right. We pretend we know what we are doing, but we don't; we can't. It is an impossible situation: we have the power to play God by prolonging or ending life, but we don't have and never will have God's wisdom.

EXPECTATIONS

I should have seen it coming. The clues were all there. In retrospect, they were more like billboards than clues.

I met them during the first summer of my residency, when I was working in the emergency room.

"*M*y name's Tory," she said.

I looked up. That wasn't the way parents usually responded when I introduced myself in the emergency room. I hadn't looked at her or the baby yet. I had just picked up the sheet of paper on the outside of the door and walked in reading it. "Eight-day-old baby girl with diarrhea," it read. "No fever."

The mother was an African-American girl who looked very young. I walked over to the stretcher where the baby lay, and she moved away. Most mothers stayed close by. I did a quick assessment of the baby before starting to ask questions; she didn't look sick at all.

I sat on the stretcher next to the baby; Tory did not move from the chair against the wall. I asked her when the diarrhea started. She gave me a vague story of slightly loose stools since birth, without fever or any other symptoms. She thought maybe it was her formula.

"Any problems with the pregnancy?" I asked.

"No."

"Was she born on time?"

"A week early."

"Any problems with the delivery or with the baby right after she was born?"

"No."

"Does she have a pediatrician?"

She shook her head. She hadn't been looking at me as she answered the questions. She stared at her hands and twirled her bracelet around and around. She was small, maybe a little more than five feet tall, plump, with hair braided closely around her head. She wore a big dark blue T-shirt, shorts, and high-top sneakers.

When we took histories of newborns, we usually asked about the mother's obstetrical history. "Had you ever been pregnant before?"

She paused and then nodded.

"What happened?"

"I had an abortion," she said quietly.

"How old are you?"

"Fifteen," she said.

I tried not to let any reaction show on my face. I rose from the stretcher and picked up the baby. "She's beautiful," I said. "What's her name?"

"Jenise." She sat and watched me with her arms in her lap, her face blank.

I did a more careful examination of the baby; she was fine. There was some stool in the diaper, but it looked en-

tirely normal. I explained to Tory as I changed the diaper
that there was nothing wrong with the baby, that newborn
babies sometimes have loose stools, and that she didn't need
to change the formula.

"Okay," said Tory. She stood, picked up the diaper bag,
went over to the stretcher, and began to dress the baby.

I watched her for a moment.

"Look, I work in one of the clinics here one afternoon a
week," I said. "Jenise needs to have a pediatrician. If you'd
like, I could give you my card."

Tory looked up at me and shrugged. "Okay," she said.

I gave her one of my cards. She stuck it in a pocket of
the diaper bag and went back to dressing the baby.

"We like to see babies for their first appointment when
they are two weeks old," I said.

"Hmm," Tory said without looking up.

I left, thinking that I would probably never see them
again.

Two weeks later, Tory and Jenise showed up in the clinic
to see me.

"I tried to get an appointment for last week," said Tory,
"but you didn't have no openings."

"That's okay," I said. "I'm glad you came."

"Hmm," Tory said with a shrug.

The baby lay awkwardly across her lap, dressed in a pink
sleeper that was much too large for her.

We talked about how things had been going. The baby
seemed to be doing well. Tory said she was really tired,
though, because the baby had her up two or three times
during the night.

"She gonna keep doing that?" she asked.

"For a while, yes."

"Shit," said Tory. She looked down at Jenise and shook
her head.

I asked about where she lived and who else lived there. She lived in an area of Boston called Roxbury, near Dudley Station, a low-income neighborhood with a fair amount of street crime. She lived with her mother and her ten-year-old brother.

"How old is your mother?" I asked.

"Thirty," said Tory. So the mother had been fifteen when Tory was born.

"Does she help you out with Jenise?"

"Sometimes."

"Does she work?"

Tory laughed. "Nah."

"Why do you laugh?"

"She's too drunk to work most the time."

"Oh," I said. I didn't know what else to say.

"She ain't drunk all the time," Tory said quickly. "Just sometimes." She looked at the piece of paper I was using for my notes. I put down my pen.

"What do you do for money?"

"We get welfare. And my mom's boyfriend, he gives us money sometimes."

"Where's your father?"

Tory shrugged. "I dunno."

"What about Jenise's father?"

"We ain't goin' out no more. He comes around, though."

"Does he help, like with money or with taking care of her?"

"He brought diapers once. You gonna check the baby, or what?"

We undressed Jenise, and I examined her. She was growing well and appeared very healthy. Tory moved away from the table again as I examined the baby.

"You're doing a good job," I told Tory.

"Hmm," she said.

I put Jenise back in her sleeper, gave her back to Tory, and sat down. I talked to her about colic and safety and other two-week-visit topics. She looked at me without expression and nodded. I couldn't tell if she was listening.

"Tory, who is your doctor?"

"I went to Brigham."

"That was for your prenatal care. Who is your regular doctor, you know, for your checkups and birth control and stuff?"

She looked confused. "I don't know," she said.

"If you'd like, I could be your doctor, too. We see teenagers here."

She shrugged.

"Think about it, anyway. You have the number to make an appointment if you want to. I need to see Jenise when she's two months old for her first set of shots."

"Okay. Bye," she said, and she was gone.

I got Tory's chart from Medical Records and spent some time reading it. I found the record of the abortion, which had taken place when she was thirteen years old. She had also been seen in the gynecology clinic twice with gonorrhea and chlamydia. Flipping through the chart some more, I found a disturbing emergency room visit three years before for a broken finger that apparently occurred during a fight with her mother's boyfriend, at least according to the social worker's note. That note said that Tory had been sexually abused by her father, who left when she was six and hadn't been heard from since.

At Jenise's two-month checkup Tory looked better. Jenise was still waking up at night, she told me, but only once. The baby was dressed in what looked

like the same sleeper she had been wearing last time. This
time, though, it fit better. Tory held her less awkwardly.

Jenise was still doing well, gaining weight and growing.
She was a cute baby, very alert; she looked around the room
and watched me as I examined her. Tory still kept her distance, but this time she almost smiled when I congratulated
her on doing a good job, and she was quick to hold the baby
when she cried during her shots.

I asked her about the broken finger.

"Oh, that was a long time ago," she said.

"Has he ever hurt you or tried to hurt you since?"

She wouldn't look at me. "I keep outta his way," she said.

I asked about school. She wasn't going, she told me. She
dropped out when Jenise was born. She saw my expression
and said quickly, "My welfare worker says there's some GED
program I can get into, though. I just gotta find day care for
the baby so's I can go. They put her on some waiting lists."

"Good," I said. "School's really important, if you want to
get a job or do anything with your life."

She shrugged. Clearly she hadn't thought much about the
rest of her life.

I asked her if she had ever used birth control.

"I can't take them pills," she said.

"Why not?"

"I keep forgettin'. I try takin' them, and then I forget for
a few days, and they're no good anymore, so I stop. They
gave me some at Brigham the other day when I went for,
you know, that checkup after the baby or whatever, but I
ain't takin' 'em."

"What about condoms?"

"My boyfriend, he don't like 'em."

"So you're going out with him again?"

She squirmed. "Sorta."

"Sleeping with him?"

She wouldn't answer, but I could tell the answer was yes.

"So what are you going to do?" I asked.

"Whaddya mean?"

"For birth control."

"Huh?"

"Tory, you've been pregnant twice already. If you don't use something, you're going to get pregnant again, and soon."

"No, I won't."

"How's that?"

"When I got pregnant with Jenise I wanted to get pregnant. I don't want to get pregnant now."

"Come on, Tory, you're not stupid. You know it doesn't work that way. What about the other time? Did you want to be pregnant then?"

She turned away and shrugged.

"And what about infections? You've had a few already. You're going to end up really sick or with scars in your tubes so you won't be able to have babies when you want to. And AIDS, too—you're putting yourself in danger of getting that."

"My boyfriend don't have AIDS."

"Are you sure?"

She was quiet.

"Look, I'm not trying to get on your case. Well, maybe I am. But I just want you and Jenise to be healthy and happy, and I don't want you to have another baby before you are ready."

Tory was quiet, sullen.

"Maybe could you try just one more time taking the Pill?"

She shrugged. "Maybe," she said.

"How many months of it did they give you?"

"Two."

"Okay. In two months if you make an appointment, I can get you more. They explained to you how to take it?"

She nodded.

"Did they give you condoms?"

She nodded again and got up.

"Jenise needs to come back in two months for her next set of shots. You can make the appointment out front."

"Yeah, right," she said, and shut the door behind her.

I really blew it, I thought. I scared her off—now she'll never come back.

Tory didn't show up with Jenise for her next appointment, and I figured that she didn't want me as a doctor anymore. I wasn't surprised, but I was sad, and I hoped that she was at least getting health care for the baby somewhere else. I tried calling the phone number entered on the chart, but the phone had been disconnected.

About a month later my beeper went off. I answered the page.

"Hey."

"Who is this?"

"Tory."

"Hi, Tory. What's up?"

"I know I missed her appointment," she said, "but I didn't have no money for the bus. She's sick—can I bring her in today?"

"What's going on with her?"

"I dunno, but she keep cryin', and she feel hot."

I looked at my watch. "I don't have clinic this afternoon, but I could see you at around two. Could you be there then?"

"Yeah."

"Do you have money for the bus?"

"I'll get it."

"Good. I'll see you then."

They were waiting for me when I got to the clinic about two-fifteen. I brought them into one of the exam rooms. Jenise was crying and leaning against Tory; she looked miserable. Tory didn't look particularly worried. She seemed annoyed and kept telling the baby to stop crying.

"How long has she been sick?" I asked.

"Few days," said Tory. "I thought she'd get better, but she didn't."

"I see," I said. She probably should have called me sooner, I thought. I took the baby's temperature; it was 102 degrees. I examined her and found that she had an ear infection, a fairly bad one. Jenise had a reason to be miserable. I went to the med room and got some antibiotics so I could give her the first dose right away, and I wrote out a prescription, which I gave to Tory.

"You need to fill this on your way home."

"I lost the baby's card."

"What?"

"You know, the Medicaid card. I lost it."

"Can you get a new one?"

"I guess so."

I went back to the med room and got enough of the antibiotic for the whole course of therapy, as well as some Tylenol. "I'll give this to you, but you have to go to wherever you need to go to get a new card by the end of the week. Okay?"

Tory looked sheepish. "Okay," she said.

"And she needs to come back in two weeks to have her ear checked and get her shots. She's behind. Make the appointment on your way out."

"Okay." She put the medicine in the diaper bag. Jenise stopped crying and looked up at Tory, who smiled at her. I hadn't seen Tory do that before.

"Next time," I said to Tory, "give me a call as soon as you think she's sick. If we catch things early, it makes it easier to treat them."

She looked at me. "All right," she said, and she sounded sincere.

I thought of asking her if she was taking the birth control pills, but I didn't want to say what I would have had to say if she said no. I'd said enough for one day.

Maybe that was part of it. I was always so careful about what I said and when I said it, afraid I would scare her away. Maybe I gave Tory the upper hand that way, or at least maybe she sensed that she could keep secrets from me. Then again, I was just the doctor, right?

*T*ory was right on time for Jenise's next checkup. The baby was coming in for her six-months' shots at eight and a half months, but all things considered, I figured we weren't doing too badly.

Jenise was wearing red overalls, a yellow turtleneck, and little yellow Reebok sneakers. I commented on how cute they were, and Tory smiled. Jenise smiled, too, and squirmed to get out of her mother's arms. Tory sat her on the floor, and Jenise pulled herself to standing by holding on to Tory's chair; she turned and grinned at the two of us, clearly proud of herself.

Tory laughed. "She just learned to do that."

Things were going well, Tory told me as Jenise sat on the floor, played with some tongue depressors that I gave her, and babbled. The welfare worker had finally found a day care placement for Jenise, and Tory was back in school. She was getting her own welfare check now, which meant less fighting with her mother over money.

"Are you taking the birth control pills?" I asked.

"Yes, I am," she said with mock indignation. "I was gonna ask you for more."

"No problem," I said, and wrote her a prescription.

We undressed Jenise over her protests, and I examined her; she was fine. Tory stayed next to the examining table the whole time. I went out to get the shots, and when I came back Tory was blowing kisses into her belly, and Jenise was giggling loudly. They didn't hear me come in, so I stood and watched them for a few moments, enjoying their game.

I gave the shots. Jenise screamed, and Tory picked her up immediately. "It's okay, baby," she said into Jenise's ear as she hugged her tightly. "It's okay."

I watched them as they left, and I felt happy. Even though she was only sixteen, it seemed Tory was learning to be a good mother. I felt more hopeful for them than I ever had before.

I think something happened to me at that visit. I became comfortable with how things were going with them, and perhaps that comfort made me less vigilant.

When I saw Jenise for her one-year checkup, Tory was quiet, distracted. I tried to engage her in conversation, but she wouldn't chat. I asked her if anything was wrong; she said no. All she said during the visit, actually, was yes and no, and that was only in response to my questions. Jenise, who had recently learned to walk, demonstrated her new skill for me and smiled. Tory watched her without expression. It worried me.

A few days later Tory called me. "Hey."

"Hi, Tory."

"Can I come today?"

"It's not my clinic day, but I can see you if it's important."

"Yeah, it's important."

"What's up?"

She said something; I couldn't make it out.

"What?"

"I said I think I'm pregnant."

My stomach sank.

"I'll see you this afternoon. Can you be there at three?"

"Uh-huh," said Tory.

As soon as she arrived, I had her give a urine sample to send to the lab for a pregnancy test. She wouldn't look at me as we sat down in the examination room.

"What happened, Tory?" I asked. "I thought you were taking the pills."

"I told ya, I can't take them pills."

"But—" I started to argue but stopped. "When was your last period?"

"I don't remember."

"Last month? The month before?"

"Before that. I don't remember, okay? Maybe June."

"Tory, that was three months ago. Are you sure?"

"No."

She got undressed, and I did her pelvic exam. I didn't need the results of the test; she was definitely pregnant. Not only was she pregnant, she was at least three months along, if not a little more, given the way her uterus felt.

She got dressed and sat on the chair next to the desk.

"You are pregnant, Tory. And not just a little pregnant, either."

"I know."

"What do you want to do?"

"I want an abortion."

I could feel myself getting tense. "Tory, if you knew you were pregnant, and you knew you wanted an abortion, why didn't you call me sooner?"

Tory was quiet for a while. "I was goin' to have it," she

said finally. "My boyfriend wanted me to. I didn't want 'nother one, but he did, so I said okay."

"What changed your mind?"

"We ain't going out no more."

"What happened?"

"He beat me up bad one night, and I called the cops, and he be pissed at me."

"He's pissed at *you?* Tory, he beat you up. Who *cares* if he's pissed at you!"

She wouldn't look at me.

"Tory, are you sure you want this abortion? You're not doing it just to get back at him or something like that?"

"No, I ain't doing it 'cause of that. I don't want 'nother baby. I never did, I told you."

It was such a delicate balancing act she was doing with Jenise and school and the rest of her life. If she had another baby, school would probably be out of the question, at least for a while. She would have to manage a toddler and a newborn at the same time, something I wasn't sure she was capable of physically or emotionally, and I couldn't see her mother stepping in to help much from what Tory had told me about her. But still . . .

"Have you thought about having the baby and giving it up for adoption? There are a lot of people out there who are dying to have a baby, who would love it and take good care of it."

"No way. I couldn't give no baby of mine up."

I felt angry and wanted to say something, but I stopped myself. She was only sixteen, with a life much harder than I could possibly imagine. Who was I to stand in judgment— and who was I to expect a sixteen-year-old to be sensible and rational?

"Late abortions like this are a bigger deal, Tory."

"That's okay," said Tory. "What I gotta do?"

"I can't send you to one of the clinics—they won't do it. You'll have to go to the Brigham, and they're going to want an ultrasound first." I picked up the phone to make an appointment for the ultrasound, then put it down. "You're going to have to tell your mother, Tory."

Tory quickly turned her head and stared at me. "No way."

"You have to. You're under eighteen. They have to have parental consent."

"I can't. No way." She covered her face with her hands.

"Why, Tory? Couldn't you talk to her, explain?"

"No."

"What would happen if you told her?"

"She'd kill me. She'd kick me out of the house."

"I'm sure she wouldn't kick you out of the house. You've got a little girl to take care of."

"Listen, you don't know my mother." She looked up at me; she was crying. "She don't care 'bout Jenise or nothing. She'd kick me out."

She turned away from me, facing the door, wiping tears off her face with the back of her hand.

"There is one way," I said hesitantly.

"What?" said Tory, still facing the door.

"You can go to court. Planned Parenthood can get you a lawyer."

She turned to look at me.

"But you have to get yourself there and dress nicely. And you have to get yourself to Brookline for the ultrasound. And you can't be late to either one, not even a little." I just couldn't imagine Tory pulling it off.

"Okay," she said.

"You really think you can do it?"

"Hmm . . ." She shrugged.

I called Planned Parenthood and arranged for her to see a lawyer. I made the appointment for the ultrasound and gave Tory directions to get to both places. With my voice shaking slightly, I called the Brigham and made the appointment for the abortion. I wrote it all down on a piece of paper for Tory, who had stopped crying and looked pretty much the way she usually did—expressionless.

She did pull it off. She paged me once from a pay phone in a subway station when she got lost on her way to meet the lawyer, but otherwise it went smoothly. She got her ultrasound, which showed that she was about fourteen weeks pregnant. She put on a dress, got to court on time, got the okay from a judge not to have her mother's permission, and showed up on time for the abortion. Never before had I seen her put so much effort into something, and never would I see it again.

I should have seen it coming. But in a lot of ways, things were going well. Jenise was turning into a bright, precocious, beautiful little toddler. Tory was good with her. She always called when Jenise was sick, and I liked Tory's manner with her daughter in the office; she seemed genuinely loving and caring. Jenise responded to her warmly, which I took as a good sign. Tory stayed in school—or so she told me.

In retrospect it should have meant something to me that I dropped my expectations significantly. Yes, Tory brought Jenise in quickly and more or less on time when she was sick, but I was still having trouble getting her in for well child care and shots. When she had a regular appointment scheduled, I didn't really expect her to show up. I would call and tell her to reschedule, and sometimes she did, but most of the time she didn't, so I incorporated the well child care and shots into the visits for rashes and sundry other illnesses.

I dropped my expectations for Tory's health care, too. She

got both gonorrhea and chlamydia; I treated them and lectured her again about condoms, but I didn't expect it to work. I gave up on oral contraceptives. I would mention it every time I saw her, but I didn't make a big deal out of it the way I had before.

She still saw the boyfriend who beat her up, and it was clear even from the little she said about him that he was a drug dealer. There were other boyfriends, too, about whom Tory said even less. When I asked if they did drugs, she acted ingenuous, said she didn't know, and seemed to agree with me when I talked about the dangers of drug use. I didn't pursue it further.

It was so gradual, so insidious. At the time, if I thought about how I had lowered my expectations, I just thought that I was learning to be realistic instead of idealistic.

I was much more surprised than I should have been when an investigator from the Department of Social Services called to ask me questions about Tory and Jenise. She told me that a 51A had been filed for child neglect against Tory, who had been found to have a significant drug problem and was in a detox program. It wasn't the first time she had been in detox, either. She had been spending most of her welfare check on the cocaine her boyfriends sold her.

Jenise was put in foster care with a family who, for convenience, preferred to take her to their local pediatrician, so I haven't seen her since. The last I heard, she was doing well. I've never met the family she is living with. The DSS worker told me they have lots of children, some theirs, some foster children, and that they live in Mattapan, another low-income area of Boston. I just hope she's getting attention and encouragement so that she's not pregnant at fifteen like her mother and her grandmother.

Tory was back with her mother briefly after the detox program, but it didn't work out. The two fought, and Tory tried to kill herself by taking an overdose of her mother's sleeping pills. She ended up in a foster home in a community south of Boston. I haven't seen her, either. When I last spoke with the DSS worker, they were having a lot of trouble with her. She was refusing to go to school and disappearing for days at a time.

I think about them often and feel very sad. I wanted to believe that everything was going to be okay for them, and I wanted to believe that I had helped them. I stopped seeing things I should have seen; I saw what I wanted to see and nothing else. Tory probably knew what I wanted to believe, and didn't want to disappoint me. So she let me disappoint her.

THE PRICE
OF HOPE

Vinnie DeAngelo sat on his hands on the chair next to the stretcher in the emergency room. He wore baggy green shorts with "Boston Celtics" printed on them, a gray T-shirt with the words *Boston Police* in small black lettering, and black high-top sneakers. His light brown hair was cut close to his head on the sides and a little longer on top; he'd put gel or something on it so that the top part stood up nearly straight. He had brown eyes with long eyelashes and a small, faintly freckled nose.

He was pale and a little thin. Besides that, at least at first glance, he looked fine. He looked like any other eleven-year-old boy.

His mother, Anna, sat on the other chair. She was of medium height, rounded but not overweight, with dark, thick, curly hair that fell to her shoulders. She looked to be in her late thirties, but her voice and her gestures made her seem younger.

I was the junior resident on call for Oncology, the cancer

223

service. I had been called down to the emergency room to admit Vinnie to the hospital.

Anna had clearly told the story many times, but she patiently told it again to me. Vinnie had been losing weight for a while, she said, and acting tired. She hadn't known what to make of it; she thought maybe he was playing sports too much, and she had tried to get him to cut back a little and go to bed earlier. Then the bruises started. She didn't think anything of them at first, thought he was just being clumsy, but then one day she looked at him when he got out of the shower, and, well, she knew something was wrong.

"Show the doctor the one on your leg, Vinnie," she said.

Reluctantly Vinnie stood up. He turned around and pointed to the back of his left lower leg. There was a big bruise there, about six by six inches, deep red and purple. There were also some smaller bruises scattered on his legs and arms.

"He's also got these little red spots, I forget what the other doctor called them," said Anna, pointing to some tiny bright red spots on Vinnie's arms.

"Petechiae," I said. They are caused by bleeding in tiny blood vessels under the skin. We see them whenever there is a problem with the body's ability to control its bleeding.

I motioned Vinnie up onto the stretcher and did the rest of his physical exam. Besides the bruises and petechiae, the only other thing I found was a slightly enlarged spleen. Anna paused for a couple of minutes, watching me, and then finished the story.

"Yeah, petechiae, that's right. So I took him to the pediatrician today. He did a blood test, and when he saw the results, he said we had to come here for more tests. So we came here, and they did more blood tests, and they're going to do that bone marrow test."

She was very matter-of-fact as she spoke, glancing frequently at her son. I knew that she knew more than she was saying. She knew, as I did, that Vinnie had leukemia. We wouldn't know what kind of leukemia until the oncologists did the bone marrow biopsy, but the story, the physical exam, and the blood test results were unmistakable.

I was brief; clearly she didn't want to discuss leukemia right then in front of Vinnie, and anyway, we needed the bone marrow biopsy results to talk about the specifics of treatment. I told them I would do the paperwork so that as soon as they were done with the bone marrow biopsy they could get out of the emergency room and up to a hospital room. I explained that one of the emergency room doctors would be putting an IV into Vinnie's arm and that they would be giving him some medicines so that the bone marrow biopsy wouldn't hurt. Once we had the results back, we would talk some more. Vinnie made a face when I mentioned the IV, but otherwise he was expressionless. He watched his mother closely. Anna kept her eyes on me as I spoke; they became red and moist. She nodded and smiled politely as I left the room.

I was thankful that I didn't have to say anything more, that I didn't have to try to explain leukemia or comfort them or tell them what was going to happen to them. I hadn't spent much time yet on the oncology service, but it had been long enough to be thoroughly depressed by the horrors of childhood cancer. The oncologists kept telling the other residents and me that we were getting a skewed view by seeing only patients in the hospital and not those who came to the clinic. You are seeing the worst of it, they told us. There are lots of success stories, lots of children who are cured and go on to live normal lives.

I wanted to believe them, but it was hard sometimes. Day

after day I was seeing beautiful children whose bodies and lives were being ravaged by cancer and its treatment. There was so much pain and suffering, and it was often drawn out and unrelenting. The oncologists quoted good rates of survival, but one child on the ward had died already that month, and there were others whose survival, at least long-term, did not seem likely.

The pediatric oncologists were an upbeat group of doctors, in general. Perhaps one needs to be so as not to go crazy working in that field. But I couldn't understand where they got their optimism. Sometimes patients who had left the ward would stop by after their clinic visits to say hello to the nurses. The nurses would go on and on about how good they looked, but they didn't look that good to me. Some were thin and pale, some heavy and bloated from chronic steroid treatment. Many wore hats or wigs to cover their bald heads. None of them looked like normal children to me; they all looked *damaged,* somehow.

Vinnie's whole family was there later when the oncologist came back with the bone marrow biopsy results. He brought the DeAngelos into the family room on the oncology ward. It was a small, windowless room with a long couch and a couple of chairs. I brought in a couple more so that everyone could sit.

Vinnie sat between his parents on the couch. His father was short, about Anna's height, with a stocky build. He had dark brown hair, a pleasant face, and big, strong arms and hands. He wore jeans and a short-sleeved white shirt.

I introduced myself to him.

"Jack DeAngelo," he said with a vigorous handshake. My hand was lost in his. "These are Vinnie's sister and brother, Maddie and Leon."

Maddie looked to be around sixteen. She resembled her mother, but she was thinner, with more defined features. Her shoulder-length black hair was teased out and held with hairspray so that it was full around her face. She wore tight black pants and an oversize T-shirt. She was sitting on one of the chairs on the other side of the room from Vinnie and her parents, with her right hand resting on Leon, who was sitting on the arm of the chair. He was younger than Vinnie, around eight or nine years old. His hair was light brown, like Vinnie's, and it fell in curls around his chubby face. He seemed scared.

The oncologist was tall and thin, well dressed, and very serious. He leaned forward on his chair and began to talk.

Vinnie had leukemia, he told them, which is a cancer of the blood system. A certain kind of cell, an abnormal cell, starts growing out of control, taking over the bone marrow where the blood is made and preventing it from making the normal cells that do all the important things blood cells do. There were different kinds of leukemia, depending on which kind of cell was growing out of control. Vinnie had acute promyelocytic leukemia.

He paused and ran his long fingers through his hair. He looked at the family, who had not reacted visibly yet, and continued. This was a particularly, well, *difficult* kind of leukemia, he told them. It tended to cause more problems with bleeding than other kinds of leukemia and was more difficult to treat.

That was gently put, I thought. "More problems with bleeding" meant that Vinnie could suddenly bleed anywhere in his body, like in his internal organs or his brain, and that alone could kill him. "More difficult to treat" meant that his chances of long-term survival were probably not very good. That he had this kind of leukemia was bad news.

Jack leaned forward. He opened his mouth to say something and then closed it again, sitting back against the couch. Vinnie looked at him and then at the oncologist. He seemed confused.

We have come a long way in this field, the oncologist told them. He talked about chemotherapy, the medicines used to kill abnormal cells. The goal would be to get rid of as many of the abnormal cells in his bone marrow as possible, to see if they could get him into a remission. Whereas with other leukemias they might wait to see what happened after that, because acute promyelocytic leukemia didn't usually stay in remission, they would probably try to do a bone marrow transplant right away if they could get him into remission.

He talked about the side effects of chemotherapy and told them a little about bone marrow transplants. All of the DeAngelos' eyes were glazed, except for Vinnie's; he didn't seem to be paying attention. He played with his shoelaces, stared at the ceiling, squirmed between his parents. Anna had her arm tightly around Vinnie. Jack's hands were clasped in front of him, and he stared intently at the oncologist. Maddie and Leon were motionless, like statues.

My beeper went off, and I left the room to answer it. A nurse was calling me to replace an IV in another patient, so I didn't go back to the family room until about twenty minutes later. The door was closed; through the window in the door I could see Jack and Anna alone in the room, sitting on the couch with their arms around each other. Anna's face was buried in Jack's chest; Jack's back was to the door. Their shoulders shook the way people's shoulders shake when they sob.

*F*or a year and a half I had been watching scenes like that one. Month after month since starting residency I had been watching parents cry. It wasn't just Oncology; every month, on every service, there were seriously ill or injured children, some of whom died. I guess I couldn't have expected anything else from a residency in pediatrics, but I never expected the effect it would have on me.

I knew I would be sad, but I didn't expect a sadness I couldn't shake, a sadness that followed me home, tainted my dreams, and made it hard to go to work in the morning. I knew I would have to keep some distance, but I didn't expect to need the distance so much, to be so afraid of connecting or even making friends with some of the patients and their families.

Not all of the children's suffering was intrinsic to their illnesses or injuries. Some of it was inflicted as part of the treatment. There were IVs, blood tests, and plenty of other things involving needles. There were breathing tubes and urinary catheters and other pieces of uncomfortable hardware we attached to or put into children. So much of it was scary for the children, from CAT scans and EKGs to the simple fact that they were away from home, surrounded by adults they didn't know and didn't trust.

Most of the time it seemed worth it. Most of the time it seemed clear that we were saving lives or at least markedly improving them with our treatments. But when the children had illnesses that were incurable or unlikely to be cured, it wasn't so clear to me. As I watched them undergo all the needles and tests and treatments, I found myself wondering why we didn't just leave them alone or at least do less to them. People talked about hope and chances and medical progress, but it just didn't make sense to me.

The DeAngelos lived in Boston's North End, an Italian community abutting Boston Harbor. Jack and Anna had been born and raised there; they had been high school sweethearts. Jack was a policeman, and Anna worked in her family's bakery, keeping the books and helping out at the counter. Maddie was a junior in high school. She was a good student, they told us, but she'd be a better one if she spent a little more time with her books and less with her friends. They usually said this with a teasing smile in Maddie's direction. Maddie would shrug and smile back. Leon was in third grade, an apparently active and boisterous child whose aggressiveness had made him the star of his soccer team.

Vinnie was in fifth grade. He hated math, loved Nintendo, pizza, basketball, and any television show that had to do with policemen; he was fiercely proud of his father. He is the easy one, they told us. He's the one who has never given us a moment's worry.

The stories they told and the way they smiled when they told them made me want to cry. Nothing could ever be the same for them without Vinnie.

Most patients get at least some nausea and vomiting with chemotherapy, but Vinnie had one of the worst cases I'd ever seen. We tried every medication we knew of to make it better, but he still vomited and vomited. He lay in his bed in his darkened room—he said that bright light made him feel worse—and as often as every few minutes when he wasn't asleep he'd sit up, reach for an emesis basin, and throw up.

Anna, Jack, and Maddie took turns staying with him. They sat on the armchair next to the bed that folded out into a cot, getting up to hand him emesis basins or help him clean up after vomiting. They brought books to read while he slept; Maddie brought her homework. But most of the time when I passed the room on my nights on call, they were just staring at him as he slept.

The walls of Vinnie's room were quickly covered with cards. Everyone in his class at school made him one. His aunts and uncles and cousins sent them. All of the neighbors sent them.

"Everybody loves Vinnie," Anna told me. "It's always been that way. He was the kind of baby everyone wanted to hold. The neighborhood kids are always coming by to ask him to play. His teacher tells me he's the most popular boy in his class."

She looked over at him. He was asleep, his legs tangled in the sheet that covered him. "It's hard to describe what it is about him," she said. "He makes people happy, makes them laugh. Comes naturally to him."

Vinnie's hair fell out. It happens to everyone on chemotherapy, and we always tell people it's going to happen. We tell them, and they see all the bald children on the oncology ward, but I don't think you can ever really prepare someone for it.

He watched his hair come out as he combed it, saw it on his pillow in the morning, and looked at himself in the mirror with such sadness. Anna and Maddie brought him baseball caps; that's what the other children who had lost their hair wore. They brought him several, trying to find one he'd like; he piled them in the corner of the windowsill. When he had to come out of his room, he put one on. When he didn't absolutely have to come out of his room, he didn't come out. He lay in bed in the darkened room, watching television for hours.

One evening Jack brought in a police jacket. It was an official jacket, clean and new.

"It's from the guys at the station," he said as he handed

it to Vinnie. "We're making you an honorary member of the force."

Vinnie grabbed it and put it on. It hung on him, accentuating how much weight he had lost, but his face was brighter than it had been in days. "I'm going to be a policeman when I grow up," he told me.

There was a little silence in the room, a pause, an awkwardness. It was brief, but it was noticeable and painful.

"You sure are, kid," Jack said finally, and hugged his son.

I knew that the oncologist met with Jack and Anna after that first night to talk more about the specifics and the statistics of Vinnie's leukemia, so I knew that they knew how serious it was. They didn't talk about it, though, at least not with us. And after that first night, I never saw them cry.

They didn't say anything when the nurses came in with the many transfusions of blood and platelets and clotting factors that Vinnie needed. When the chemotherapy killed off so many of Vinnie's normal cells that it was hard for him to fight infections and he started having fevers, terrible fevers, they were very calm. They watched the nurses giving antibiotics, and they kept a cool washcloth on his forehead.

They were almost businesslike, taking their shifts and making their arrangements, and they were always pleasant. They didn't ask many questions about the chemotherapy or other treatments we were giving Vinnie. The only thing they asked questions about was the bone marrow transplant. When would we know if we could do it? Exactly what did Vinnie's blood test results need to show? When could we start testing all of them to see if anyone could be a donor?

It worried me that they seemed so fixated on the bone marrow transplant. I worried that they were using the hope of a transplant as an excuse not to face the reality that Vinnie would probably die.

Leon hardly ever came to the hospital, and when he did

he sat on a chair in the corner and never said anything. Whenever I saw him he was certainly not the boisterous child they had described. I asked Maddie about it.

"There was a kid in his class last year who had some kind of cancer and died," she said. "Leon's convinced Vinnie's going to die. It's really creepy, but sometimes he even talks about him like he's already dead."

She said it evenly, without emotion, tossing back her hair. She didn't seem like the girl they had described, either; she was very serious, and I noticed that she spent many Friday and Saturday nights in the hospital instead of going out with her friends. She seemed to watch Anna closely whenever she was with Vinnie, and her voice, her gestures, and her manner were becoming more and more like her mother's.

"I think it's just 'cause he's little, you know?" she said. "He doesn't understand about these things."

I didn't know what to say, especially since I didn't understand about these things, either.

After he got the police jacket Vinnie went out of his room more, wearing the jacket and a Red Sox baseball cap. He didn't go far, just out in the halls of the ward or to the activity room to play video games with the other children wearing baseball caps.

He was thin, haggard, and even paler than he had been that first night in the emergency room. He moved slowly and hesitantly, as if unsure that his legs would support him, unsure that his body would do what he expected it to do. He looked down or away, as if trying to slip by unnoticed.

But there were moments, usually when he was playing video games or joking with his father, when his face would light up and his frail body would become charged with energy. In those moments I could see what he had been, what he could be, and it made my sadness deepen.

At the end of my month on the oncology service, Vinnie wasn't much better. He wasn't any worse, but I was disappointed. I had been hoping for some kind of improvement, some sign that he was going to be okay. The oncologists weren't discouraged, but I was.

I went back to the ward to visit the DeAngelos a few weeks later when I had some free time during a night on call. Jack, Anna, and Maddie were all there with Vinnie in his room, playing gin rummy. They greeted me warmly; they all seemed in a good mood. Vinnie had been able to go home for a few days the week before, they told me. He was in now for more chemotherapy. The last bone marrow test had shown he wasn't going into remission, but there were less of the bad cells, and he hadn't needed a transfusion of anything in almost two weeks. Jack and Anna figured that he'd go into remission soon, and they'd be able to do the bone marrow transplant.

Vinnie sat cross-legged on the bed in pajamas and the Red Sox hat, staring at his cards. Fluid and medication dripped into him from a bag hung above his bed through clear, thin tubing that ran into an IV. He was so thin that he was almost skeletal, and when he looked up at me his eyes were dull and sunken in their sockets.

He looked like death to me. I lied, saying I had work to do, and left quickly. I hated that I was leaving like that, that I didn't stay and try to be brave with them, but my bravery was all used up.

I ran into Anna a couple of months later in the hospital lobby. She told me that Vinnie was in remission, and that when they did the tests on everyone in the family they found out that Maddie was a perfect match, so they were going to go ahead with the bone marrow transplant.

I was so surprised, I was speechless.

She went on, telling me about the plans and how excited they were. I listened and nodded, feeling happy for them and yet embarrassed. I was embarrassed because I hadn't expected Vinnie to get this far and because I didn't entirely share her enthusiasm about the bone marrow transplant. It was an amazing technology, but the time I'd spent working on the bone marrow transplant unit had been very upsetting for me.

High doses of chemotherapy are used to empty out the bone marrow so that it can accept the transplanted bone marrow, and this wreaks havoc on the patient's body. And because the bone marrow is being wiped out, the patient has almost no defense against infection, since that's where the cells that fight infection are made. So the children are put in special sterilized rooms with airflow designed to blow germs out. Visitors have to scrub their arms and hands as if they were surgeons about to do an operation, and they have to wear special gowns and masks. The children can't leave the rooms, and there are strict rules about who and what can enter them.

It was just so hard to watch. The children were miserable and so isolated. The nurses and the social workers worked with the families to try to make the weeks or even months more bearable, but it was a hard job.

The children changed. Their skin often grew darker, and their faces became different. They never looked like the pictures taken of them before they got sick. Their personalities changed, too. Some kept their spirits up, but most grew very subdued.

Despite all the precautions, there were inevitably fevers;

we would give antibiotics and hover and worry. There was so much to worry about with bone marrow transplants: the side effects, the blood tests, the fevers, whether or not the new bone marrow would "take," and if it did, whether the patient would get "graft versus host disease," a serious complication of the whole process. And even if the transplant took and everything went well, there was always the chance that the cancer would come back.

The oncologists seemed to minimize these worries. The important thing, they said, was that these children had a chance for a cure.

It should have made sense, and they said it with such confidence, such assurance. And not all the children had a difficult time. But when I scrubbed, gowned, and masked and went in to see the ones hot with fever, with rashes on their skin and their mouths filled with sores, huddled under their sheets in their sterile little prison cells, I sometimes wondered if it was a chance worth taking.

I wanted to visit Vinnie while he was on that ward, but I never did. I wanted to know how he was, and I even started walking over there a few times, but I always stopped before the big doors. Vinnie was the first child with cancer whom I had met at the very beginning, before treatments transformed his body or his spirit. It upset me to think about him going through a bone marrow transplant, and I was afraid to see what had happened to him. I was having enough trouble making it through the days as it was.

About six months after the bone marrow transplant, I met Anna and Vinnie on the street outside the hospital. I didn't recognize Vinnie; it wasn't until I saw Anna that I realized who he was. Steroids had made him much heavier, with very full cheeks, and his skin was darker. He still had freckles, but they were a different color and larger. His hair had grown back coarse and a deeper brown. His eyes seemed smaller, and dulled somehow.

Anna greeted me with a grin. The transplant was a success, she told me. Vinnie had been home for a long time. They had just come from a checkup at the clinic.

"So far, so good," she said. "Doesn't he look wonderful?"

My first thought was that "wonderful" wasn't the word I would have chosen. But then it dawned on me, so clearly that I was ashamed I had not understood before.

He was alive, and he had a chance to keep living. It might not be a good chance, but at least for now he was with his family, and he could play Nintendo, eat pizza, play basketball, and watch all the policeman shows he wanted.

Suddenly my mind was filled with images of Vinnie and his family. I felt the persistence and purity of his beauty and their love for him, things I had not let myself feel before. And in that moment a little bit of my bravery, and my hope, came back. This time what we had done made sense, and realizing this made my sadness suddenly much lighter.

"Yes," I said. "He does look wonderful."

THROUGH A
MOTHER'S
EYES

I woke up a little after six. The early morning sunlight leaked around the blinds into my hospital room,
brightening the quiet air. I sat up slowly; the drugs I had
been given the night before were wearing off, but I still felt
dizzy and weak.

My husband was asleep on the armchair he had pulled
up close to the bed. I reached over and touched his arm. His
eyes flew open, and he sat up quickly, his expression
alarmed.

"I'm okay," I said. "Could I see her?"

He smiled and left the room.

The night before, I had given birth to my first child. She
was much larger than anyone expected—ten pounds, five
ounces—and the delivery had been difficult. My skin and
muscles tore as she came out, and I lost a lot of blood. I
heard her cry right after she was born, a loud, vigorous cry
that told me she was fine. Right then, that was enough for
me. I was in too much pain and too disoriented from the
anesthetics and the blood loss to even really look at her. It

took the doctor more than an hour to sew me up, and then I was taken to the recovery room, where I fell into an uncomfortable sleep. The hours after that were a blur.

Mark came back into the room, pushing a bassinet made of clear plastic. He brought it over to the bed and then reached in, lifted out the baby, and handed her to me.

Michaela filled my arms as I cradled her and stared at her incredulously. Her eyes were closed; she had soft dark hair, long eyelashes, a tiny nose, and perfect pink lips. I unwrapped the blanket so that I could touch all of her: her belly, her feet, her hands, and her long, delicate fingers. As I played with her fingers she woke up and clasped my finger, and her deep blue eyes looked into mine.

What I felt in that moment was more powerful than anything I expected. I was stunned by the reality of this child in my arms, by the incredible miracle that she had actually grown inside me. I was stunned by the kind of love I felt for her: instantaneous, deep, and total. In that moment my entire world rearranged, and she became its center.

M ichaela Evelyn Brown, named for my father and my grandmother, was born in February of my senior year of residency. It was hard to arrange a maternity leave given the constraints of the residency schedule, and I had to go back to work full-time when she was seven weeks old. I cried every day during the last week of my leave. To comfort myself, I tried to concentrate on the fact that there were only three months left of residency. Somehow, I thought that being separated from my baby for many hours at a time was going to be the only hard part about being a mother and a doctor at the same time. I was wrong.

The emergency room was full of its usual noise and bustle when I arrived for my first shift back. It was early evening, and the waiting area was full of parents and their children, some running around and some huddled miserably in the parents' laps. I went through the big doors, past the busy secretaries, and down the corridor to the charting area where the doctors and nurses did their paperwork and made their phone calls. I felt nervous, although I wasn't sure why.

I passed a few residents. Two smiled hello, the others just nodded at me, intent on whatever it was they were on their way to do. I was surprised; I'd expected a different response to my return. I'd had a major, life-altering experience. Wasn't anyone going to congratulate me or at least ask how I felt?

Then again, I realized, residency itself is a major, life-altering experience. Childbirth doesn't pale in comparison, but it becomes less impressive.

John, the senior I was relieving, looked tired and seemed anxious to leave. I followed him along the corridor from exam room to exam room as he ticked off the patients and their diagnoses and what still needed to be done for them. It was the senior's job to oversee these things, along with arranging admissions and helping the medical students and interns.

"Room twelve is a little kid with fever," he said quickly, in a businesslike tone. "Not real sick. Thirteen is a urology patient with what looks like a post-op infection. We're waiting for the fellow to come down. Fourteen is a wheezer . . ."

It was all so familiar to me, the diagnoses and the tests and the treatments, but it wasn't immediate and comfortable as it had been before. Before, I was just a doctor, and my world was relatively narrow, defined by predictable routines. Before, my responses and actions came easily. Now that I was a mother, everything felt off kilter.

Shortly after John left, a medical student came up to me.

He was tall and skinny, with dark hair and glasses, wearing a white coat with overfilled pockets. He introduced himself as Louis and asked if I was the senior; I said yes. He asked if I would help him draw blood from a two-month-old baby he was seeing. He'd done it before, and he was pretty sure he could do it by himself, but he wanted someone in the room with him in case he had trouble.

I followed him over to the exam room and listened as he explained to the mother of the baby that although the baby didn't have a fever, it would be a good idea to do a blood test to be sure that her fussiness wasn't caused by an infection.

The mother was in her early twenties, with short brown hair and pale skin. She swayed back and forth slightly, holding the baby girl against her shoulder. The baby's face was turned toward the mother's neck, and her eyes were open. One hand was touching the mother's neck, and the other grasped a fold in her shirt. As the mother swayed she rubbed the baby's back, gently, rhythmically. I felt a rush of recognition. This was how I so often held Michaela.

Ada, the nursing aide, came in and reached to take the baby, to bring her to the treatment room. Slowly, reluctantly, the mother gave the baby to her.

I had never been so aware of a patient's mother before. Parents had always been important, of course, but they were a secondary issue. We concentrated on the children and considered the parents' reactions and feelings later, if we had time, and even then there was often a perfunctory quality to our conversations and explanations. There was nothing necessarily wrong with this, but now that I knew what it felt like to be a parent, I wished I'd paid more attention to them.

Louis was waiting for me, ready to go to the treatment room. I put my hand on the mother's shoulder.

"She's going to be okay," I said. "We'll bring her right back." The mother looked at me with reddened eyes and tried to smile politely. My heart ached for her.

In the treatment room, Louis took out a needle and syringe and tubes to collect blood. Ada laid the baby on the stretcher and sang one of her Puerto Rican lullabies as Louis tied the tourniquet around the baby's arm. She was a lovely little girl, chubby and fair-haired, with blue eyes just like Michaela's.

Louis looked over his shoulder at me. I came closer, so I could watch what he was doing. His movements were a little awkward, but not incorrect. I watched him feel for a vein and then put the needle through the baby's skin.

The baby started to cry, a screaming, desperate cry. It ripped through me; I felt actual pain in my chest, and tears rushed into my eyes. As I looked at the baby I suddenly saw Michaela lying there instead. The pain in my chest grew worse, my heart beat quickly, and I could feel myself starting to tremble. I had never felt this way before.

Louis didn't look at me, and I was glad. He concentrated on the needle, moving it deeper and in different directions, trying to find the vein. I prayed that he would find the vein quickly. If he didn't, I was going to cry, and I didn't want to cry in front of him.

He found the vein; dark red blood rushed through the tubing into the syringe as he pulled back on the plunger. It seemed an eternity before the syringe was full and he took the needle out of the baby's arm. Quickly Ada put on a Band-Aid, scooped up the baby, and left the room.

Louis looked at me. He seemed calm and pleased with himself.

"Good job," I said, wondering if my voice sounded as shaky to him as it did to me.

He turned to clean up, and I left the room. I walked

briskly to the back hallway, went into the staff bathroom, and locked the door behind me.

I stared at myself in the mirror. I looked the same as I ever had. There was nothing different about my face or my hair or my hands. If anything, I looked more the same now that my stomach was flat again.

But I didn't feel the same. I felt like a completely different person, and I felt awful.

I leaned against the bathroom door, trying to relax and collect myself so that I could go back out and do my job. I am simply out of practice, I told myself. I just need a little time. I will get used to this again.

Not that I'd ever been used to it. I had never been able to get used to watching children suffer, and my sadness had never lifted completely. But I had coped; I had managed to keep my composure in front of other people, do my work, and come back the next day. I coped by separating myself and my emotions from the work as much as possible.

I developed strategies to help me separate. I found it helpful to concentrate on the science, on the intricate and interesting pathophysiology of the disease rather than the child lying in front of me suffering from it. The culture of residency encouraged this. When we discussed patients we often referred to them by their diagnoses rather than their names. We talked about "the wheezer," "the bronchiolitic," "the meningitic," "the rule-out sepsis," and on and on. We discussed the tests and medicines and theories and then, almost as an afterthought, the child.

When sticking needles into children, I found it helpful to concentrate intensely on my technique. I would do the procedure as quickly, efficiently, and elegantly as I could. I would stare only at the part of the body I was working on, shutting out the cries of the child, never looking at his face.

Whenever I had trouble separating, I took comfort in

thinking about how I was part of the medical profession. I had great faith in medicine. It seemed full of miracles. We could look inside the brain with magnetic resonance imaging, inside the womb with ultrasound. We could even look at genes and predict who would get certain inherited diseases. There were medicines to do almost anything imaginable, from helping the heart beat, to improving moods, to curing infections and many kinds of cancer. Babies could be conceived in petri dishes and, if born too early, kept alive with special machines. Hearts, lungs, livers, and kidneys could be transplanted, offering a second chance to people who would otherwise die. Medicine was powerful, and being part of it made me feel powerful.

When I became a mother, everything changed. My strategies for separating simply didn't work, because I saw Michaela's face in every child and imagined myself in the place of every parent. When I heard a child cry I heard Michaela's cry instead, and all I wanted to do was hold and comfort the child. I didn't want to finish putting in his IV, I didn't want to discuss his disease. I couldn't concentrate on the science or the procedure. All I could think about was the child.

I no longer felt powerful, either. I hadn't lost my faith in medicine, but I looked at it differently.

I had always known that medicine had limitations. I knew that not every illness could be cured and that some patients die. But in the context of all medicine's miracles, its limitations seemed reasonable and not overwhelming. Once I became a mother, the limitations became overwhelming. It didn't matter to me how many miracles medicine had produced. It couldn't guarantee me my child's health and well-being, so it would never be miraculous or powerful enough.

At night, after work, I would hold Michaela in my arms,

rocking her, in the soft darkness of the bedroom. It was as if the world would disappear or at least stop for a moment because there was nothing, nothing else but me and this baby, my daughter. Her eyes would close and her breathing quiet and her little body would relax and nestle into mine as she eased into sleep. I'd hold her for a while, not wanting to put her down. As I looked down at her tiny, perfect face, I would be overcome by love for her and by terror that something might hurt her or take her from me. I hated that as a doctor I knew all the things that could happen, and I hated that I had to face them every day at the hospital.

Within a week after my maternity leave ended I knew that I had made the right decision in choosing to do primary care pediatrics after residency. I couldn't stay in a hospital setting, especially not a tertiary-care hospital filled with the sickest of sick children; it had simply become too painful. I wanted to be out in a clinic or office doing the kind of pediatrics I liked best: helping children and their families stay healthy and happy and building relationships with them. After all, the only thing I can truly guarantee the parents of my patients, besides that I will be conscientious and careful, is my relationship with them. I can't guarantee that their children will always be well, but I can guarantee that no matter what happens, I will do everything I can to help.

I have two children now. My son, Zachary, was born eighteen months after Michaela. As I hold the warm blessings of their bodies next to mine, I know that the real miracles in this world don't have much to do with science or technology.

In a moment, a child is conceived. He grows inside his mother and is born, in a rush of pain, fluid, and blood. He continues to grow, learning and exploring, adapting and changing. He learns to eat and to call for his mother, to walk and to talk, to hate and to love. He finds his place in the world and makes his connections, strong or weak, with the people around him.

These, I think, are the real miracles: the miracles of everyday life and everyday people, miracles so ordinary that their wondrousness often slips by unnoticed and unappreciated. The way a baby calms in his mother's arms. The way we can speak without words, in a gesture, a smile, a purposeful silence. The small acts of kindness that make such a difference: an offered hand, a lost wallet returned, a secret kept. That we fall in love and build families. That we find the courage to take risks. That we exist at all.

I think now that the real miracles of medicine lie not in its scientific component, but in its emotional component. Medical science has produced some amazing things, but now I think that they aren't so much miracles as important discoveries figured out by very smart and industrious people. They are explainable and reproducible, which to me makes them wonderful but not miraculous.

The emotional component of medicine holds the mysteries of life and humanity that we will never figure out. Why, for instance, do some patients get better and some don't, even when they have the same illness and receive the same treatment? We tend to attribute it to the illness; we say that the patient who did poorly had a particularly malignant form of the cancer or a particularly strong strain of the virus, or whatever. But I think it has more to do with the patients themselves: their spirit and strength, what they have to look forward to, what and whom they believe in, how well they are loved. There is an entire dimension to illness and health that will never be explainable or reproducible, no matter how smart we are or how industriously we study it.

The faces, the voices, and the moments: I chose to go into medicine because of them, so that I would be surrounded by them. Now, as a mother, I know why even more clearly. There is nothing more beautiful, miraculous, or important than people, their relationships, and their stories.